MEDICINAL HERBS
of EASTERN CANADA

MEDICINAL HERBS
of EASTERN CANADA

Text and art by
BRENDA JONES

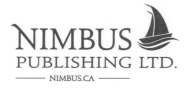

NIMBUS
PUBLISHING LTD.
—— NIMBUS.CA ——

Nimbus Publishing Limited
3660 Strawberry Hill Street, Halifax, NS, B3K 5A9
(902) 455-4286 nimbus.ca

Printed and bound in Canada
NB1460

Editor: Emily MacKinnon
Cover Design: Heather Bryan
Interior Design: Brenda Jones & Rudi Tusek

Library and Archives Canada Cataloguing in Publication

Title: Medicinal herbs of Eastern Canada : a pictorial manual /
art and text by Brenda Jones.
Names: Jones, Brenda, 1953- author, illustrator.
Description: Includes bibliographical references and index.
Identifiers: Canadiana (print) 20200165038 | Canadiana (ebook)
20200165046 | ISBN 9781771088626
(softcover) | ISBN 9781771088633 (HTML)
Subjects: LCSH: Medicinal plants—Canada, Eastern—Identification. |
LCSH: Herbs—Therapeutic use—
Canada, Eastern. | LCSH: Herbals—Canada, Eastern. | LCSH:
Naturopathy. | LCGFT: Field guides.
Classification: LCC QK99.C3 J66 2020 | DDC 581.6/3409713—dc23

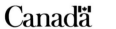 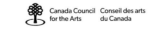 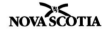

Nimbus Publishing acknowledges the financial support for its publishing
activities from the Government of Canada, the Canada Council for the Arts,
and from the Province of Nova Scotia. We are pleased to work in partnership
with the Province of Nova Scotia to develop and promote our creative
industries for the benefit of all Nova Scotians.

*To Merlin,
for his patience and support over the last
few years as we trekked through ditches,
fields, and marshes, swatting mosquitoes
and gathering plants*

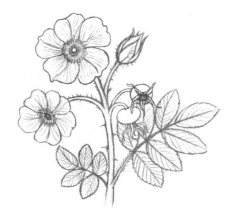

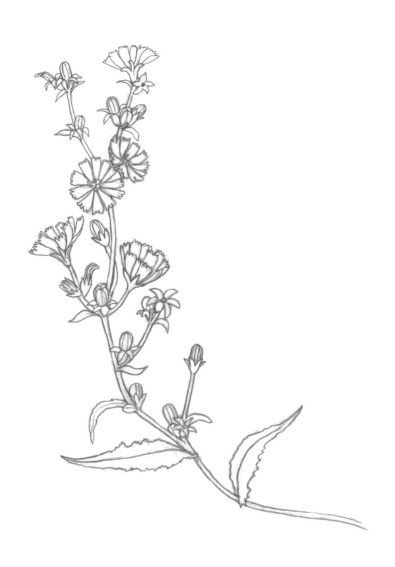

TABLE OF CONTENTS

ACKNOWLEDGEMENT

*Many thanks to the people of Eel River Bar
First Nation in northern New Brunswick
for sharing their knowledge, teachings,
and ceremonies.*

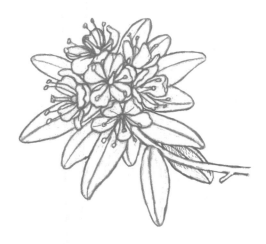

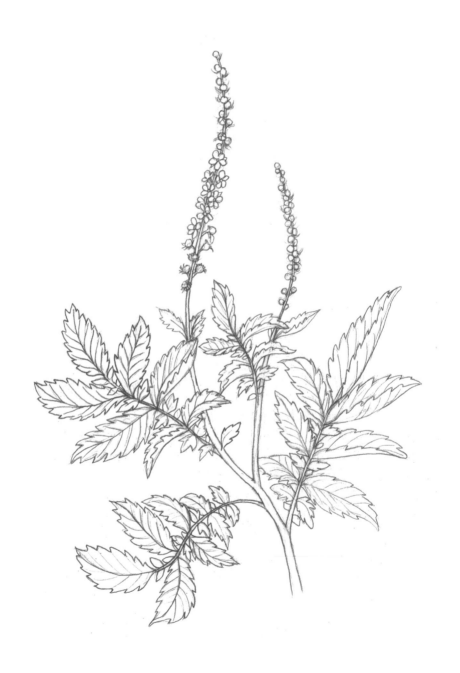

INTRODUCTION

Ever since ancient times herbs have played a major role in healing in all cultures throughout the world. Traditional remedies were passed down from one generation to the next, using local plants and trees to cure disease, heal wounds, or ease pain. Shamans, healers, and midwives played an important role in society, particularly in Indigenous cultures, and their knowledge was gifted to future generations through word of mouth so as not to lose these important medicines. Unfortunately, much of this knowledge has since been lost, mostly in the last hundred years, due to the takeover of modern science and the pharmaceutical industry, attempted genocide of Indigenous cultures, and destruction of rare species and their habitats. However, there has been a resurgence of interest in medicinal herbs recently as people are dealing with more and more chronic disease and finding little relief in pharmaceuticals. Although they will always play a major role in the medical industry, drugs are not the only answer; there is much room for a more gentle, holistic approach to healing, and for working with nature and all the gifts the earth has given us.

I first developed an interest in plants as a young girl when my mother and I would take off into the woods for an afternoon with our tin pans to create fairy gardens. We amassed all sorts of mosses, Ground Spruce, Indian Pipes, Teaberries, Mayflowers, Violets, and bright-coloured toadstools, arranging them into the tiny pan gardens along with a few rocks and sticks. When we brought them home they were set up on our front step or amongst the Hollyhocks to attract any magical creatures that may pass by in the night. Although it was the time spent with my mother that I keep close to my heart, I also appreciate how she passed on her love of the forests and flowers. Nature has been a source of grounding and comfort for me ever since, whether through planting my own garden and digging my fingers into the sweet-smelling, loamy soil, or just through taking walks by myself in the countryside. There is a healing energy in the earth, and the farther we are away from it, the more disconnected we are from our own souls.

I spent the first twenty years of my life on Prince Edward Island, a place vibrant with a healing energy that easily seeps into every pore when you spend any time in the great outdoors. I think I only learned to truly appreciate the beauty of Atlantic Canada after I spent thirty years in a big city; sometimes we can only understand what we had when it is no longer there. During my time in Montreal, I was so focused on earning a living and bringing up my daughter that I failed to recognize my body was craving the ocean and the peace and safety of cool forests and open fields. I longed for the place where I could see the horizon and the stars, watch the sun rise and set, and observe storms rolling in towards the land. I would often drive for two hours just to escape the noise and pace of the city, only to find that hundreds of other people had decided to do the same thing. My short visits to the Island were never enough to fully recharge my batteries, and by the time I was in my fifties I was burnt out and had chronic insomnia and digestive problems. I knew I had to make a permanent change.

That change came in the form of a cottage on the south shore of PEI, a little piece of paradise, with 360 degrees of horizon, perched on the red cliffs of the Northumberland Strait. It was there that I began to reconnect with my roots and find a sense of balance. I was surrounded by wildflowers, so every day I would roam the fields and shores, collecting bouquets and shells. Before long, I developed an interest in knowing the species I was finding. I amassed stacks of herb books and researched plants online. I soon realized many of these plants were medicinal and could possibly help with my health issues. This led me to creating binders full of information cut and pasted together, and soon I was experimenting with tinctures and salves and my kitchen was full of drying herbs. I knew I had found a new passion.

It wasn't until I moved back to the Island permanently that I started to see the potential for putting together a book on herbal medicines. All the books I had found dealt with European or American species—often unavailable in our Maritime climate—and it was frustrating trying to identify anything from the tiny photos in the field guides. After mistaking Cow Parsnip for Angelica once (fortunately, I had not tried to pick it, as it probably would have caused severe dermatitis!) I resolved to create my own illustrations. This was not a big stretch for me, as I have been illustrating children's books and making a living as an artist for most of my life. Before I knew it, I had a couple of dozen drawings completed and realized I was well on the way to making a book. My publisher loved the idea and I loved the thought of spending so much time with these amazing plants, but it never occurred to me that it would take me the better part of five years to complete—although I've enjoyed every minute of it.

At this point in my life I can't call myself an herbalist, because I believe that title belongs to those who have dedicated their lives to understanding herbs and using them to heal others. It takes many years of study of the properties of plants, knowledge of how the body works, and, according to true herbalists, understanding the subtle energies of each species and how they interact with our own energy on a deeply personal level. My real goal with this book was to create detailed pictures of the herbs available in Atlantic Canada to facilitate identification for amateur collectors, and to give the average person an over-view of their properties and how to use them.

But there is so much more to learn, most of which is not available in books.

I found this out at a workshop I attended at a reserve in northern New Brunswick, where the healers impressed upon us the importance of intuition and dreams in healing, and the necessity of healing the soul before the body will heal. We have become so accustomed to the ways of allopathic medicine, taking a pill to make us feel better, that we've forgotten the depth of our spirit; we've forgotten that we are more than just flesh and blood. We can list all the traditional medicinal uses of each plant, and over time and in the right dosage they will probably help ease certain symptoms, but we need to realize that those symptoms are a message that there needs to be a change. If this message is not heeded, our bodies will send us louder and more serious messages until we pay attention.

We are complex creatures, all with different makeups and metabolisms, and what may work for one might not work for another. Understanding the energy of the body and knowing the language of the plants requires a keen intuition that takes time to develop. But we are all capable of learning it if our minds are uncluttered and our intention is clear. Our con-nection with the earth has withered and frayed over the last hundred years, particularly for those living in cities. We have become fearful of all things wild, including our own inner wildness.

This became clear to me one day as I was visiting a friend who had just moved to the suburbs of a major city. Her house had a large backyard, still partially wild and unmown, and while exploring it I came across a patch of wild Strawberries growing amongst the weeds. I picked a big handful—while simultaneously stuffing my face—then promptly went inside to offer her the rest. She looked at me incredulously and said, "Oh, no, I can't eat those; I don't know what they are!" Even with my reassurances, she would not taste them.

It struck me then just how disconnected our society has become from Mother Nature. How sad that she had lost that trust, that she was so afraid of something as basic as a wild Strawberry, yet she would have no problem eating a package of Strawberries wrapped in cellophane, shipped from thousands of kilometres away, grown under unknown conditions and undoubtedly sprayed with chemicals. How sad that she would never know that sweet burst of flavour, untouched by humans and packed full of vitamins and sunshine. We've lost so much in this sanitized, plastic-wrapped world of ours! Children who have never visited a farm have no idea where food comes from, and adults living in the city couldn't survive without a supermarket down the street. Our minds have been poisoned by TV shows and movies of people who have ventured into the wilderness only to be chased by vicious creatures, or swimmers who are torn apart by monsters hiding just below the surface of the ocean. Is it any wonder people are so afraid of nature?

Yet, research shows that immersion in nature is not only pleasurable, but also highly beneficial for our health and well-being. Studies coming out of Europe have found that people who spend at least two hours per week in green spaces are both healthier and happier than those without this contact. It can lower blood pressure, reduce anxiety and stress, improve immunity, and just make us feel better. I am hoping that this book will encourage you to get out there with your family and do some "forest bathing," and to pay attention to all the amazing plants you'll discover on your journeys.

Since I began researching this book, I have started my own backyard garden and now have thirty or more edible herbs, some of which I planted, and some of which have mysteriously appeared and made themselves at home over the years. Some are weeds that I welcome in and then regret doing so as I watch them take over, but all are tasty and nutritious. My salads during the spring and summer months include many wild-crafted plants found either in my yard or within a thirty-kilometre radius: nutty-tasting Watercress, crunchy Purslane, Dandelion greens, Borage flowers, Violets, lemony Sorrel leaves, spicy Mustard greens, Mint...and maybe even a few wild Strawberries!

It is important to note that if you are wild-crafting your herbs, you must be conscious of where you pick them from and how abundant they are. Never use herbs that are growing along busy highways, next to farmers' fields that are sprayed with pesticides, or anywhere near land that may be contaminated. Always use plants that are healthy-looking and strong, not eaten by insects or diseased, and make sure there are enough plants left behind that you won't be depleting the local population. Only take what you need, and if you are using the top of the plant, don't disturb the roots; this way, it can grow back. If there are only a few, or the species is endangered, leave them be. I have gotten into the habit of leaving a pinch of tobacco each time I take something from its environment; it reminds me that the plants are a gift and we should leave something in return. Indigenous peoples have always been conscious of this, giving thanks for everything that is taken from the land; it is never taken for granted or wasted. We would all be better off learning from these teachings.

I should also emphasize the importance of being sure you have correctly identified any plant before consuming it. I have tried to include as much detail as possible to assist with identification, because I want people to feel confident and comfortable using plants for healing. For this reason, I have also included a section at the end of this book (see page 155) to help you to identify the most common poisonous plants. I urge you to consult it when gathering herbs or foraging in the wild and to teach your children which ones to avoid. A plant may be medicinal in small doses, but there are some that can become toxic if used for too long, in doses larger than what is recommended, or by using a different part of the plant, so please be aware of and heed the warnings provided.

Spending time in the great outdoors can be so enriching, opening our minds and senses to the many gifts our world has to offer, and, when done with care and respect, it can teach us a great deal about ourselves.

Disclaimer

The information provided in this book is intended for educational purposes only. Every effort has been made to ensure the accuracy of this information through extensive research, botanist and Indigenous consultation, and proofreading, however I make no guarantees regarding errors or omissions and assume no legal responsibility for injuries resulting from the use of the remedies in this book. The suggestions included are not intended as a substitute for professional medical care.

HERBAL PREPARATIONS

These are some of the most common methods of preparing herbs.

INTERNAL REMEDIES

| INFUSIONS |

Probably the simplest way of using herbs, infusions are simply teas made from a herb or group of herbs in order to extract the healing properties. This method is best for the leafy parts and flowers of the plant, and they should be chopped fine to expose as much surface as possible. Since fresh herbs contain more water, we usually double the amount. A standard infusion consists of:

- 1 tsp. dry (2 tsp. fresh) herbs
- 1 cup boiling water
- Let infuse for 10–15 minutes, preferably in a covered teapot, particularly if the herb is fragrant, to keep in the volatile oils. Strain into a cup and drink hot or cool.

| DECOCTIONS |

This method is used for more woody parts of the herb, like stems, bark, roots or rhizomes, and sometimes berries. They require a bit more steeping to extract the medicines, and should be chopped as finely as possible before decocting.

- 1 tsp. to 1 tbsp. fresh or dried herbs, chopped or ground finely
- 1 cup cold water
- Place in a pot, cover, and heat on the stove until it comes to a boil. Reduce heat and simmer 20–40 minutes. Cool slightly and strain. You may make a larger batch, but leftovers should be refrigerated and used within 48 hours.

| TINCTURES |

Tinctures are made by macerating fresh or dried herbs in 80-proof alcohol, preferably vodka or brandy, or other solvents like apple cider vinegar or glycerine. This extracts more of the medicinal qualities and preserves the herbs much longer than if they were simply dried. The standard method for making alcohol tinctures is:

- Choose enough fresh or dried herbs to fill a Mason jar about ⅔ full. Make sure they are clean and dry, and chop or grind to increase surface exposure to the alcohol.
- Pour in enough alcohol to completely cover the plant material. As the plants will increase in volume, you may need to add more alcohol later. Cover with lid and place in a cool, dark place for about 6 weeks. Shake the bottle every couple of days.
- After the 6 weeks, strain the mixture into a measuring cup or bowl covered in several layers of cheesecloth. Gather up the cloth with the plant material in it and squeeze out as much of the liquid as possible to extract the maximum amount, as this is where it is more concentrated. Let settle and strain again through a sieve if necessary. Pour through a funnel into amber dropper bottles, label and date, and store in a dark cupboard.

| SYRUPS |

Syrups are a good way to make herbal decoctions more palatable, particularly if they happen to be strong and/or quite bitter. The sweetener, usually sugar or honey, also helps preserve the medicine for a longer period of time. Here is a basic recipe for a cough syrup:

- ⅓ cup dry herbs
- 2 cups cold water
- ½ cup honey or sugar
- Place woody herbs or roots and water in a saucepan and bring to a boil (if you have leaves or flowers, add them at the end of simmering time). Allow to simmer until liquid has reduced by about half. Cover the pan and let sit for an hour or so. Strain out the plant matter and return liquid to the pot. If adding honey, heat very gently, just enough to soften the honey, and remove from heat. If sugar is added, heat just long enough to dissolve the sugar. If you wish, you can add up to 3 tbsp. of brandy or other alcohol.

EXTERNAL REMEDIES

| INFUSED OILS |

Herbs can easily be infused into oils for use as massage oil, to relieve itchiness, soreness, or inflammation, or as a bath oil. We typically use organic cold-pressed virgin olive oil, but almond, grapeseed, or coconut oils can also be used. They will last up to a year if kept in a cool, dark place.

- Make sure herbs are clean and dry. If using fresh herbs, do not wash them, as you want the least amount of water possible in the jar. Leave them out on the counter for a few hours to let bugs escape, then chop and pack into a sterilized Mason jar, up to ¾ full.
- Cover with oil, leaving ½ inch at the top, making sure plant material is completely submerged. Use a knife to release any air bubbles in the liquid. Cover with wax paper and screw on lid. Leave the jar in a sunny window for about 2 weeks, shaking occasionally.
- Strain into a bowl covered with cheesecloth and squeeze out any remaining liquid. Place strained liquid into a clean, dry jar. If you used fresh herbs, let the jar sit for a day or two to see if any water settles in the bottom. Pour into an amber bottle, making sure any water stays behind, and store the oil in a cool dark place.

| OINTMENTS OR SALVES |

These are a great way to protect and soothe inflamed skin and to heal sores or wounds. They contain oils or fats but no water, so they form a layer on top of the skin rather than sinking into it like a cream. Any kind of infused oil may be used in this basic recipe.

- 20 grams beeswax
- 100 ml. herb-infused oil
- 1 small (120 ml.) Mason jar, sterilized
- Gently warm the beeswax and oil together in a double boiler or Pyrex bowl set into a pan of water. When wax has melted, place a drop on a saucer and place in the freezer for a minute to test the consistency. If it's too hard, add a little more oil, if too soft, add a little more wax. Remove from heat, cool slightly, and add 10–20 drops of essential oil if desired.

| LINIMENTS |

A liniment is basically a mixture of a strong herbal decoction and alcohol, which is readily absorbed into the skin to relieve the pain of sprains, sore muscles, or broken bones. The addition of alcohol adds to the shelf life of the decoction, and aids absorption of the herbs. The basic recipe is:

- 1 part vodka or rubbing alcohol
- 2 parts decoction (should be well strained before adding the alcohol)
- You can also make a good liniment by placing a mixture of herbs in a sterilized jar and adding enough Witch Hazel or rubbing alcohol to cover. Screw on lid, and let the mixture sit for 4–8 weeks. Strain and pour into a sterilized bottle or spray bottle and label to remind you that it is NOT to be taken internally. It will keep for about a year.

| POULTICES |

A poultice consists of solid fresh plant material that has been mashed or bruised to release the medicines, or dried herbs that have been ground and made into a paste by adding warm water. This paste is placed directly on the skin, and can be covered with a hot water bottle if desired. They are usually made from warming and stimulating herbs, vulneraries, astringents, or emollients.

| COMPRESSES |

Compresses or fomentations are clean cloths like gauze or cotton which have been soaked in a hot infusion or decoction. They are placed on the affected area and kept as hot as possible to enhance the action of the herbs. A hot water bottle can be placed on top of a compress to keep it warm for a longer period of time. Vulnerary herbs, stimulants, and diaphoretics make good compresses.

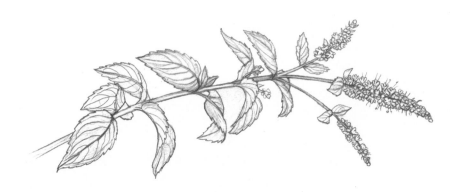

AGRIMONY

Agrimonia gryposepala
Agrimonia striata

FAMILY: *Rosaceae* (Rose)

OTHER NAMES: Tall Hairy Groovebur, Woodland Agrimony, Grooved Agrimony, Cocklebur, *Fr.* Aigremoine

PARTS USED: Aerial, in bloom

CHARACTERISTICS: Cool, drying, bitter, slightly sweet, and sour

SYSTEMS AFFECTED: Digestive, liver/gallbladder, urinary, kidneys

ACTIONS: Astringent, alterative, antibacterial, tonic, diuretic, vulnerary, cholagogue, hepatic

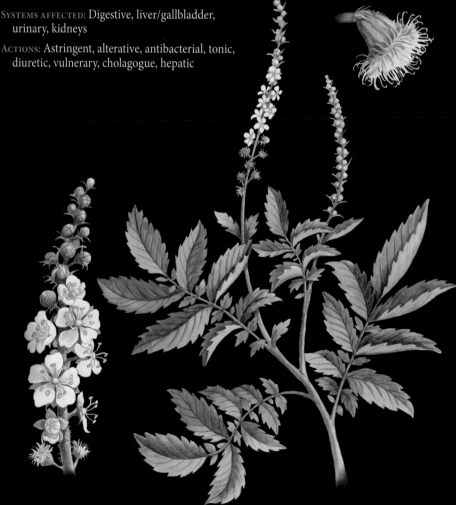

Agrimony actually consists of several different species that grow in eastern Canada, typically in woodlands, around the edges of fields, and along roadsides. Once called "Fairy's Wand," it is a native perennial, which grows to a height of 120–180 cm., and has an erect, hairy stem with alternate compound leaves composed of many unequal leaflets, smooth above, hairy underneath, and strongly serrated. The tiny yellow 5-petalled flowers are slightly aromatic and grow on slender-branched erect spikes, which bloom between July and September. The fruit are seeds with little hooks that attach themselves to anything that passes by—usually animal fur. The upper stems of the plant should be gathered early in the summer and dried in the shade, not above 40° C.

MEDICINAL USES:

Liver problems, indigestion, diarrhea, wounds, urinary infections

- Contains tannin, so its bitter, astringent properties stimulate the liver and increase digestive secretions, flushing out toxins. It relieves symptoms of diarrhea and mucous colitis, indigestion, gallbladder inflammation, jaundice, and gout. Its action on the liver may relieve other symptoms of liver congestion such as dry, brittle hair, dysmenorrhea (menstrual cramps), or (in Chinese medicine) inner anger or frustration.
- Infusion makes a good spring tonic.
- Eases urinary inflammation and cystitis, kidney pain and stones.
- Gargle is antibacterial and soothes mucous membranes, eases sore throat, laryngitis, and mouth ulcers.
- Ointment or infusion from seeds and leaves used topically can help heal burns, slow-healing wounds, inflammation, or varicose veins and bruises. Stems external bleeding.
- May be effective in lowering blood-sugar levels, but more study is needed.
- Weak infusion soothes eye irritation.

FOLKLORE: When placed under a person's head at night, Agrimony was said to induce a deep, dreamless sleep.

INFUSION: Add 1 cup boiling water to 1 tsp. dried herb, infuse 10 minutes. Drink 3 times a day until symptoms dissipate.

TINCTURE: 1–3 ml., 3 times a day.

IMPORTANT: Do not exceed recommended dosage. Do not use if pregnant or breastfeeding. Patients with excessive bleeding should use with caution. May cause photodermatitis.

ANGELICA

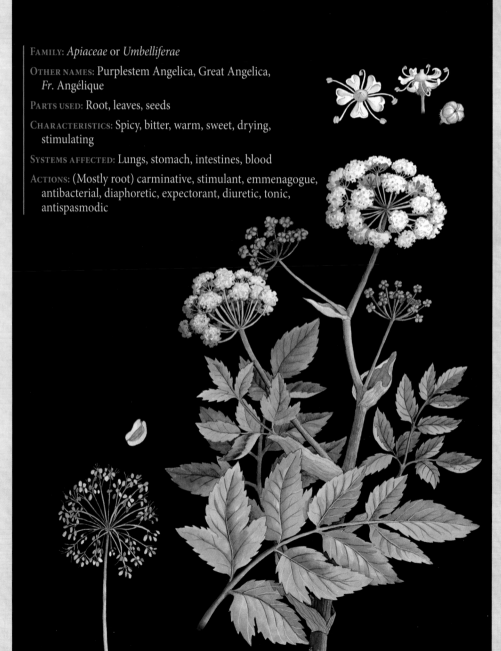

Angelica atropurpurea

FAMILY: *Apiaceae* or *Umbelliferae*

OTHER NAMES: Purplestem Angelica, Great Angelica, *Fr.* Angélique

PARTS USED: Root, leaves, seeds

CHARACTERISTICS: Spicy, bitter, warm, sweet, drying, stimulating

SYSTEMS AFFECTED: Lungs, stomach, intestines, blood

ACTIONS: (Mostly root) carminative, stimulant, emmenagogue, antibacterial, diaphoretic, expectorant, diuretic, tonic, antispasmodic

A member of the carrot family, this large, robust perennial resembles its European relative, *A. archangelica*, not only physically, but medicinally, although it is perhaps not quite as potent and is less aromatic. Its hollow, purplish stems often grow up to 1.8 metres tall. The leaves are also on hollow footstalks, which are covered in a sheath at the base, and are composed of numerous bipinnate leaflets with finely toothed edges, the veins ending on the tips of the notches. The yellowish-green to white flowers are grouped into large round umbels and pleasantly aromatic. Dig roots up in the fall of the first year, slice longitudinally to speed drying, and store in an airtight container. Angelica is most potent when tinctured in alcohol. Collect leaves in early summer before flowering.

Since this plant, along with others in the carrot family, closely resembles Woodland Angelica, Poison Hemlock, Water Hemlock, Cow Parsnip, and Giant Hogweed—all of which are highly toxic—it is imperative to correctly identify the plant before even touching it! Do not harvest if any of the above are growing in the area.

MEDICINAL USES:

Rheumatic complaints, digestive weakness, gas, menstrual irregularities, coughs and colds

- A warming herb, Angelica acts as an expectorant, and helps relieve symptoms of colds, flu, bronchitis, and other upper-respiratory complaints where there is a thick, sticky mucus and unproductive cough that requires soothing. It relaxes the cough reflex and encourages the production of loose, thin mucus that is more easily coughed up. Promotes perspiration.
- Tea stimulates appetite and digestive process, as it encourages gastric and pancreatic secretions; helps with anorexia. Relieves gas, heartburn, flatulence, stomach upsets, and colic.
- Poultice of mashed roots warms and stimulates circulation, and helps with gout, arthritis, and rheumatism, as well as swelling and pain from broken bones.
- Tea balances female hormones, relieves menstrual cramps, eases the symptoms of menopause, brings on menstruation (but is not to be used when pregnant).

OTHER USES:
- Young shoots and stems are sweet and can be cooked or eaten raw.
- Essential oils from seeds and root are used in perfumes and as flavouring for gin, vermouth, and Chartreuse.

FOLKLORE: Angelica was given its name in 1665, by a monk who claimed he dreamt of an angel who told him the plant had the power to prevent and cure bubonic plague. It has always been purported to have special powers against poison, plague, and contagious diseases, and is said to ward off evil spirits and spells and prolong life. A decoction mixed with bathwater is said to remove negativity and hexes.

TEA: 1 tsp. powdered seed, dried root, or leaves per 1 cup boiling water. Steep 10–15 min.

COUGH SYRUP: Boil 2 tbsp. root in 4 cups of water for 3 hours. Strain and add honey. Take 2 tbsp. as needed.

IMPORTANT: Not for use during pregnancy—can cause miscarriage. Avoid getting juice of the plant into eyes. Use gloves to handle. Do not use fresh roots; they must be dried. Can increase photosensitivity. Avoid if you are diabetic, as it can increase blood sugar. May increase blood clotting, so avoid if you are at risk of stroke.

BARBERRY

Berberis vulgaris

FAMILY: *Berberidaceae*

OTHER NAMES: Pipperidge bush, Jaundice berry, *Fr.* Épine-vinette

PARTS USED: Bark of root (most concentrated) or stem, berries

CHARACTERISTICS: Cool, bitter, berry
· is sour

SYSTEMS AFFECTED: Liver, gallbladder

ACTIONS: Cholagogue, alterative, anti-inflammatory, anti-emetic, laxative, hepatic tonic, antibacterial

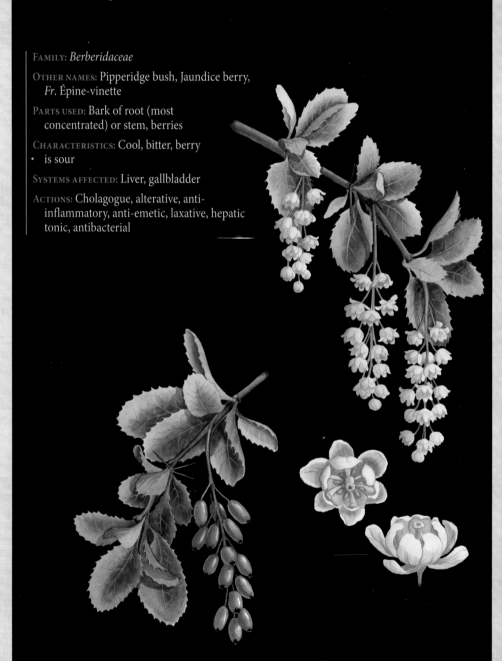

B arberry is native to Europe but grows throughout northeastern Canada. It is a bushy, deciduous shrub, about 2.5 metres high with woody smooth stems, grey bark, three-pronged spines, and yellow roots. Leaves are alternate or in rosettes, and spoon-shaped with spiny notches and prominent veins on the underside. Flowers bloom between May and June and are small, pale yellow, and grow in pendulous clusters at the tips of the branches. The red, oblong berries appear in the fall, about 1 cm. in length. It can be found along field fences and in pastures. Harvest berries and root bark in the early fall; pare off the bark and dry roots in the shade before using.

MEDICINAL USES:

Liver problems, menstrual irregularities, skin diseases, arthritis

- The yellow wood and flowers of barberry have historically been effective in treatment of liver and gallbladder problems. Used as a liver tonic, it stimulates bile production and treats inflammation of the gallbladder, stones, hepatitis, and jaundice.
- Root bark contains berberine, which is effective as an antibacterial and immune system stimulant, and is astringent—good for treating diarrhea and dysentery. Once used in a syrup mixed with fennel seed as a remedy against plague, it is an effective immune stimulant, and may help ward off infectious diseases.
- Fruit is astringent and is rich in vitamin C. The juice made into a syrup helps ease a sore throat.
- Tea made from the root bark and stems can treat stomach ulcers and indigestion.
- Supports the urinary system by relieving inflammation, infection, and discomfort.
- May lessen the symptoms of rheumatism, arthritis, and sciatica.
- Can be used externally as an eyewash, or as a gargle to treat sore throat and gingivitis.
- Some research suggests it may be effective in treating leukemia and other forms of cancer. May also improve abnormal lipid levels and high blood pressure, and may even prevent or treat diabetes, but more research is needed.

OTHER USES:
- Indigenous peoples used (and continue to use) the bark and stems to dye animal skins and fabrics.
- Berries are pleasantly acidic and can be eaten raw, or cooked in jams or jellies.

DECOCTION: Put ½ tsp. bark into 1 cup of cold water; bring to a boil. Simmer 10–15 minutes. Let steep 5 minutes. Add honey, as it is quite bitter. Drink 1–3 ounces, up to 3 times a day.

IMPORTANT: Avoid use during pregnancy or breastfeeding. Not for children under 2 years of age. May be harmful in large doses, so do not use for more than 7 days at a time, and wait at least a week between uses.

BAYBERRY

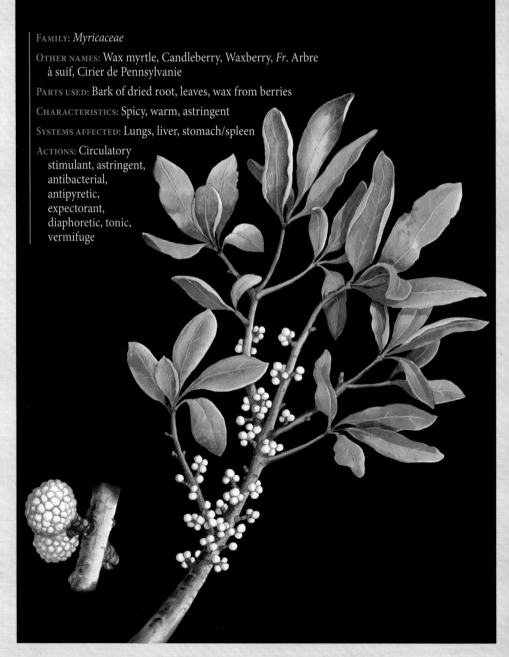

Myrica (Morella) pensylvanica

FAMILY: *Myricaceae*

OTHER NAMES: Wax myrtle, Candleberry, Waxberry, *Fr.* Arbre à suif, Cirier de Pennsylvanie

PARTS USED: Bark of dried root, leaves, wax from berries

CHARACTERISTICS: Spicy, warm, astringent

SYSTEMS AFFECTED: Lungs, liver, stomach/spleen

ACTIONS: Circulatory stimulant, astringent, antibacterial, antipyretic, expectorant, diaphoretic, tonic, vermifuge

Bayberry is a perennial native bush that grows abundantly along shorelines and near swamps and marshes. Anywhere from 1 to 3 metres tall, it has lance-shaped leaves, which are shiny and resinous, and fragrant when rubbed. Along the stems are small light-grey berries, which are covered in an aromatic waxy substance. The root should be harvested in spring or fall, the bark removed and dried before using, and stored in a dark container.

MEDICINAL USES:

Colds, flu, fevers, astringent for hemorrhoids, circulatory stimulant, sore throat, inflamed gums

- Works to rally the body's defenses against disease, especially as a decongestant, in colds, sinusitis, flu, and fever.
- Astringent, it works to stop diarrhea, mucous colitis, dysentery, and expel worms. Also for minor bleeding as in bleeding gums and excessive menstruation.
- Good for circulation in the digestive tract; stimulates bile production, helps jaundice and bowel inflammation.
- The Mi'kmaq crush the roots to a powder and use it as a poultice, a tea for arthritis and rheumatism, and as a mouthwash. The leaves have been used as a poultice for bleeding, hemorrhoids, and varicose veins. European settlers believed it could "expel wind" and ease aches and pains from colds, flu, and indigestion.

OTHER USES: Berries can be boiled in water to separate the waxy coating, which can then be used to make fragrant candles.

DECOCTION: Steep 1 tsp. of root bark in 2 cups of boiling water for 30 minutes. Add honey if desired. Will induce perspiration and improve circulation. Do not exceed 2 cups per day.

IMPORTANT: Emetic in large doses. Avoid use if you have a history of stomach or colon cancer, kidney disease, or high blood pressure. Do not use if pregnant.

BEARBERRY

Arctostaphylos uva-ursi

FAMILY: *Ericaceae*

OTHER NAMES: Crowberry, Foxberry, Hog cranberry, Kinnikinnick, *Fr.* Raisin d'ours

PARTS USED: Leaves, stems, fruit

CHARACTERISTICS: Bitter, astringent, cool

SYSTEMS AFFECTED: Heart, kidney, bladder, small intestine, liver

ACTIONS: Diuretic, urinary antiseptic, astringent

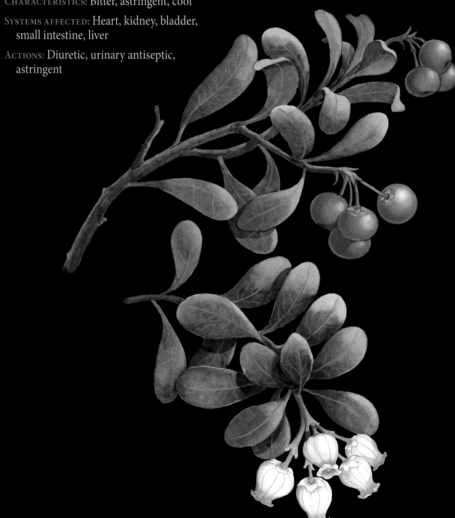

This low-growing native evergreen shrub probably earned its name, *uva-ursi*, which means "bear's grape," from the fact that bears find the berries tasty whereas people consider the flavour unpleasant. Growing to a height of about 20 cm., its trailing branches are short, woody, and covered in a pale-brown bark. The shoots are slightly hairy and rise upward from the stems. The leaves are leathery and spoon-shaped, dark green on top and paler underneath, with a coarse network of veins. The flowers appear in drooping clusters in June, each one urn-shaped, usually white, and sometimes with a reddish lip. Berries appear in the fall and resemble a small red currant. Bearberry grows in dry open woods, in gravelly or sandy soil. Collect leaves in September or October, and only in fine, dry weather when the dew has evaporated, taking only green, unblemished leaves. Dry in the sun if possible; if not, use a warm, well-ventilated shed that's free of moisture.

MEDICINAL USES:

Cystitis, headaches, wounds, general tonic

- This herb is a natural diuretic and has been a traditional treatment for bladder and urinary tract infections for hundreds of years. It is also a powerful astringent, soothing and tonifying the entire urinary system. The leaves contain a natural, potent antibiotic, which works best if the patient is on a vegetable-based diet where the urine is alkaline. Works to relieve cystitis, gravel, and other inflammatory diseases of the urinary tract.
- Traditionally used by Indigenous peoples, the stems of Bearberry and Blueberry can be infused and drunk as a way to prevent miscarriage and aid in recovery after childbirth.
- Has been used in folk medicine for years as a headache remedy. The leaves are dried and smoked, producing a mild narcotic effect.
- Salve made from the fruit can speed healing when applied to wounds.
- Protects the stomach from harmful bacteria.
- Often used in an Indigenous smoking mixture called kinnikinnick.

OTHER USES: Contains tannins, which can be used for tanning leather.

INFUSION: Mix 1 ounce of dried leaves with 1 cup boiling water. Steep 10–15 minutes, drink 3 times a day.

ALCOHOL INFUSION: Soak leaves in brandy or vodka for up to 1 week, and then add 1 tsp. soaked leaves to 1 cup of boiling water; steep 10–15 minutes.

TINCTURE: 10–20 drops, 3–4 times a day.

IMPORTANT: May cause nausea or constipation if taken in large quantities. Prolonged use may cause stomach and liver problems. It can be used when pregnant to prevent miscarriage or treat a urinary tract infection, but it may cause nausea if not taken in the right dose, so it is advisable to consult a professional herbalist. Do not give to children.

BEDSTRAW

Galium palustre (Marsh bedstraw)
Galium aparine (Cleavers)
Galium triflorum (Fragrant bedstraw)
Galium labradoricum (Northern bog bedstraw)

FAMILY: *Rubiaceae*

OTHER NAMES: Cleavers, Goosegrass, Gripgrass, Catchweed, *Fr.* Gratteron, Gaillet jaune

PARTS USED: Aerial, fresh or dried

CHARACTERISTICS: Bitter, cool, slightly dry, salty

SYSTEMS AFFECTED: Bladder, gallbladder

ACTIONS: Diuretic, alterative, anti-inflammatory, aperient, mild astringent, febrifuge, tonic, vulnerary

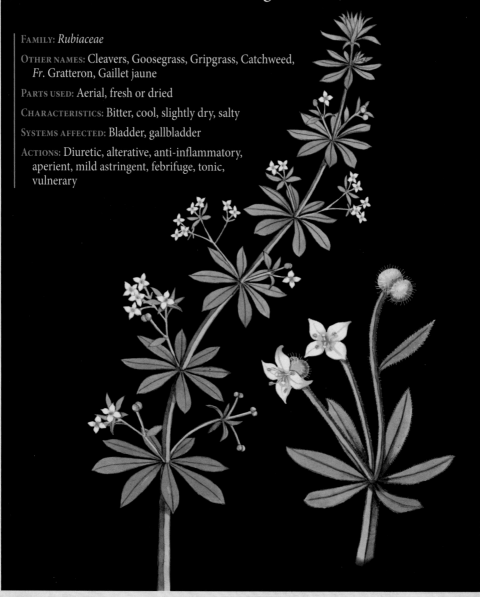

Plants in the genus *Galium* are found all over the world, and comprise over 3,000 species. There are at least seven different ones growing in the Maritimes, but the one most often used for its medicinal properties is *G. aparine*, or Cleavers. These plants are slender, angular weeds with tiny lance-shaped or oval leaves arranged in whorls around the stem, and small flowers that are white, greenish, or yellow. The plants grow in matted masses by attaching themselves to other plants and objects with their hooked bristles on the stalks and leaves. The flowers grow out of the axils of the leaves and are followed by little seedpods that are also covered in bristles and stick to anything that passes by, especially animal fur. Gather in May or June; may be hung in the shade to dry for later use, but best when the fresh herb is used, either in tinctures or infusions.

MEDICINAL USES:

Urinary infections, enlarged lymph glands, skin inflammation, insomnia, hypertension

- Juice from the fresh herb is recommended as a diuretic and blood purifier, in bladder infections where there is painful urination, and for stones. Rich in vitamin C. Cleanses and decongests the lymphatic system and kidneys.
- Infusion of the dried herb has a soothing effect for people with insomnia, and it induces a restful sleep.
- Reduces swelling and heat and drains lymph glands; helps tonsillitis, eases head colds and swollen glands. May be combined with Echinacea or Calendula.
- Crushed herb or fresh plant juice can be used as a poultice for sores, blisters, burns and scalds, psoriasis, ulcers, and insect bites. May be used in ointments and can be combined with Yellow Dock and Burdock for skin problems.
- Diuretic properties make it useful for lowering blood pressure.

OTHER USES:
- Can be used as a potherb when picked in the spring.
- Some use it as a hair tonic, claiming it makes hair grow longer.
- A red dye can be obtained from the root.
- When juice is applied daily it may fade freckles.
- Roasted seed may be used as a coffee substitute.

INFUSION: Add 2–3 tsp. dried herb to 1 cup boiling water; strain to remove bristles. Take 3 times a day, 1 hour before meals.

TINCTURE: 2–4 ml., 3 times a day.

IMPORTANT: Juice may cause dermatitis in sensitive people. Filter to avoid throat irritation. Avoid ingestion if you have a tendency towards diabetes.

BLOODROOT

Sanguinaria canadensis
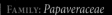

FAMILY: *Papaveraceae*

OTHER NAMES: Red root, Snakebite, Sweet Slumber, Bloodwort, Puccoon, Tetterwort, *Fr.* Sanguinaire

PARTS USED: Dried rhizome

CHARACTERISTICS: Bitter, acrid (in small amounts: drying and cooling; in large amounts: warming and stimulating)

SYSTEMS AFFECTED: Lungs, heart, liver, blood

ACTIONS: Expectorant, stimulant, alterative, antibiotic, abortifacient, diuretic, emmenagogue, febrifuge, antispasmodic, diaphoretic, emetic in large doses

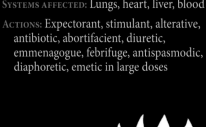

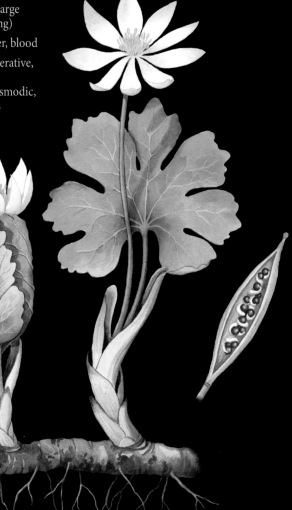

This low-growing native perennial is a powerful medicinal herb that has been used by Indigenous peoples for centuries—but it can be extremely poisonous if not used correctly. It's identified by its orangey-red rhizome, which is 2.5–10 cm. long with orangey-red rootlets, and oozes a red juice when cut open, hence its name.

Found in woods and clearings, it can grow up to 25 cm. tall, usually having only one large leaf with several lobes. In early spring, when the flower first sprouts from the rhizome, it is wrapped in a pale-green, lobed leaf. The leaf opens and a beautiful, waxy, white flower with golden stamens emerges, usually only lasting a day or two. The seedpod appears late in the summer and contains shiny bright-red seeds, which have a worm-like substance attached to each one. When the seeds are thrown out of the pod, this substance attracts ants. The ants then carry the seeds back to their nests, which are often far from the mother plant—the perfect place for a new plant to sprout up.

Please note: Bloodroot is endangered and should be cultivated, not collected in the wild. The root should be dug up in the fall after the leaves die off, then dried quickly or it will deteriorate.

MEDICINAL USES:

Bronchitis, pneumonia, skin cancer, heart palpitations

- Bloodroot is rich in alkaloids, one of them being sanguinarine, which is antibacterial, anti-spasmodic, anti-fungal, and expectorant. It also raises blood pressure and increases respiration, so it should be used with great care and only in small doses.
- Expectorant for coughs with excessive mucous production, such as pneumonia, chronic bronchitis, asthma, or laryngitis. Especially effective if there is burning and/or itching of mucous membranes.
- Improves circulation in the body; prevents heart palpitations.
- May be applied externally as a tincture, powder, paste, or ointment for skin problems like athlete's foot, ringworm, sores, eczema, skin tags, or warts. Some studies have found berberine, one of Bloodroot's components, may be effective in preventing skin cancer when exposed to UVB rays. May cause burns if used in large quantities or over a long period of time.
- Extracts added to toothpaste can treat gingivitis and prevent plaque.
- The Mi'kmaq once used it to treat tuberculosis, also as an emetic, expectorant, laxative, and emmenagogue. The juice can be used as body paint and to dye clothes.

DECOCTION: ⅛ tsp. dry powdered root per 1 cup of boiling water.

TINCTURE: 1–2 drops topically or mixed with water as a mouthwash.

IMPORTANT: Bloodroot is toxic in large doses or with prolonged use. May cause nausea and vomiting, burns to the skin and stomach, vertigo, tunnel vision, or glaucoma. Do not use if pregnant or breastfeeding. Use only with extreme caution.

BLUE FLAG IRIS

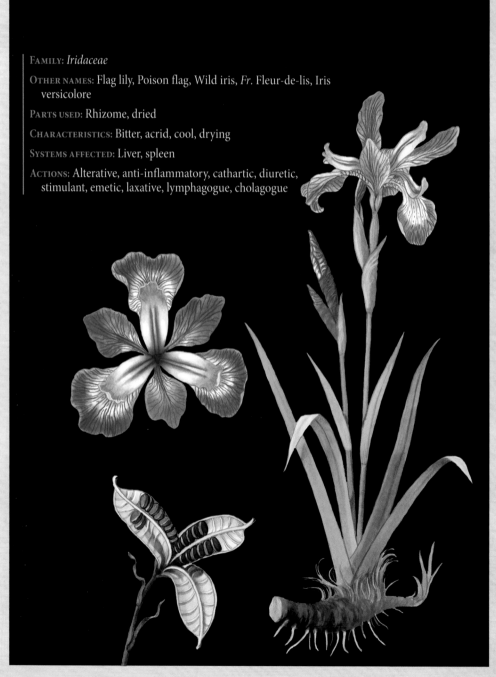

Iris versicolour

FAMILY: *Iridaceae*

OTHER NAMES: Flag lily, Poison flag, Wild iris, *Fr.* Fleur-de-lis, Iris versicolore

PARTS USED: Rhizome, dried

CHARACTERISTICS: Bitter, acrid, cool, drying

SYSTEMS AFFECTED: Liver, spleen

ACTIONS: Alterative, anti-inflammatory, cathartic, diuretic, stimulant, emetic, laxative, lymphagogue, cholagogue

This perennial indigenous plant is 0.5–0.9 metres high, and can be found growing along shorelines and wetlands. It has narrow sword-shaped leaves and during the early summer months produces pretty blue or purple flowers with yellow and white markings inside. The fleshy horizontal root has annual joints and a slight odour along with a pungent, acrid taste and should be a light pinkish-brown colour inside. Avoid using roots that are dark or reddish brown inside.

Dig up roots early in the fall, slice transversely, and dry for later use. Take care not to confuse Blue Flag with Sweet Flag, as they look very similar before the flower blooms.

MEDICINAL USES:

Liver congestion, glandular congestion, hepatitis, jaundice, various skin diseases

- Works primarily to correct problems associated with liver congestion, such as hepatitis, jaundice, constipation, indigestion, and skin problems. Stimulates bile production, and relieves stagnation in the liver and spleen. Helps treat hepatitis and jaundice. Caution: use only in small doses as it will cause diarrhea and vomiting in large amounts and should not be used if the body is in a weakened state.
- In small doses and repeated at short intervals, it stimulates the glandular system and lymphatics where there is stagnation or enlargement. Used for enlarged thyroid, enlarged spleen, or swollen lymph nodes.
- Chronic skin diseases like herpes, acne, psoriasis, eczema. Works through the liver to detoxify and purify the blood.
- Has been used by Indigenous peoples to induce vomiting in cases of food poisoning.
- Roots can be boiled in water and mashed to make a poultice to treat pain and swelling, or to relieve rheumatic joints.

OTHER USES:
- Flowers can be made into an infusion which can be used as a litmus test for acids and alkalis.
- Leaves can be dried and used to weave baskets or mats.
- Some Indigenous peoples have been known to carry the root as protection against rattlesnakes, although that would not be a problem in Atlantic Canada.

IMPORTANT: USE WITH CAUTION. Blue Flag's rhizomes are poisonous and can cause vomiting and diarrhea in large doses. Fresh root is an irritant and can cause burning in the mouth and mucous membranes. Should only be used dried and only under supervision of a certified herbalist. Do not use if pregnant or breastfeeding.

BONESET

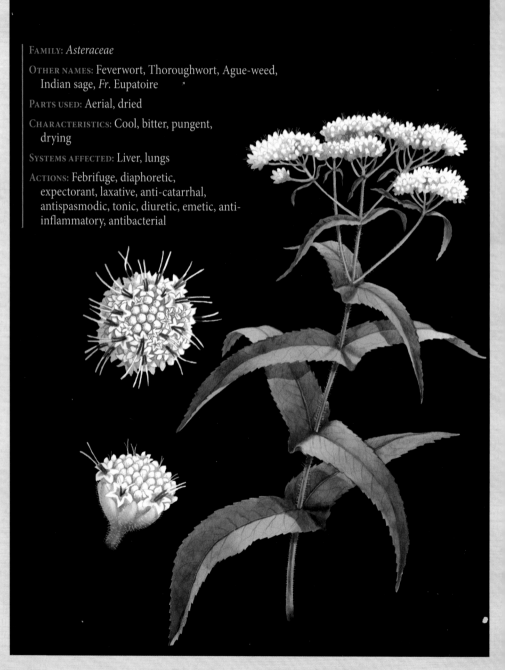

Eupatorium perfoliatum

FAMILY: *Asteraceae*

OTHER NAMES: Feverwort, Thoroughwort, Ague-weed, Indian sage, *Fr.* Eupatoire

PARTS USED: Aerial, dried

CHARACTERISTICS: Cool, bitter, pungent, drying

SYSTEMS AFFECTED: Liver, lungs

ACTIONS: Febrifuge, diaphoretic, expectorant, laxative, anti-catarrhal, antispasmodic, tonic, diuretic, emetic, anti-inflammatory, antibacterial

Boneset is native perennial that has always been popular in North America, both among Indigenous peoples and European settlers, as a remedy for that deep-seated ache in one's bones at the onset of a flu or cold. It has an erect, hollow, bristly stem 0.6–1.2 metres high, branched at the top with large, opposite leaves at right angles to the ones below, which are united at the base and appear to be pierced through by the stem. They are lance-shaped and tapered to a point, the edges finely toothed with fine hairs on the underside. The slightly aromatic flowerheads consist of 10–20 white, hairy-looking florets that bloom from July through September. It can be harvested after the flowers open, but because the fresh herb contains a toxic chemical called tremerol, it should always be used dried, as this neutralizes the toxin. It is usually found along streams and marshes and prefers wet ground.

MEDICINAL USES:

Achiness from colds and flu, intermittent fever, nervous stomach, rheumatism, arthritis

- Stimulates white blood cells to fight viral and bacterial infections such as cold and flu, promotes sweating, clears mucus congestion, and treats intermittent fever and chills. Stimulates the immune system and loosens phlegm. Good for any damp congestion in the body, such as bloating, indigestion, fluid retention, or chronic sinus congestion. General tonic, it promotes sleep. Given in small doses, it improves the appetite and aids in recuperation.
- Diuretic and laxative, it soothes and relaxes the stomach and aids in regurgitation and stomach disorders of nervous origin, aids bile secretion and liver detoxification.
- Relieves aches and pains of rheumatism and arthritis.
- Named in the nineteenth century as a cure for dengue fever (sometimes called "breakbone fever"), which causes intense muscle pains. Claims have been made that it helps treat malaria and heal broken bones, although neither has been proven.
- The Mi'kmaq use it to treat stomach ulcers and colds, and to promote sleep.

TINCTURE: 6–12 drops, 3 times per day.

INFUSION: For chills and fever: ½ tsp. (or less) dried leaves per cup of boiling water. Steep 5–10 minutes. Drink up to 3 cups per day. It is intensely bitter so you may want to add honey. If you feel nauseous while drinking it, stop—that's your body's way of telling you it's enough. Not much is needed to get the full effect. Combines well with Echinacea, Elder flowers, and Liquorice root. For stomach disorders, use a cold infusion.

IMPORTANT: Do not use as a fresh herb; should be dried before use. Should not be used if you are pregnant or breastfeeding. Do not take in large doses or over extended periods of time. Not recommended for people with liver diseases.

BURDOCK

Arctium lappa
Arctium minus
Arctium tomentosum

FAMILY: *Asteraceae*

OTHER NAMES: Lappa, Beggar's buttons, *Fr.* Bardane

PARTS USED: Root (chronic conditions), seeds (acute disorders), and leaves

CHARACTERISTICS: Bitter, slightly sweet, cool, drying

SYSTEMS AFFECTED: Kidney, liver, gallbladder, skin, blood

ACTIONS: Alterative, diuretic, demulcent, diaphoretic, nutritive, mild laxative, tonic, vulnerary, relaxant, antibacterial, anti-fungal, carminative

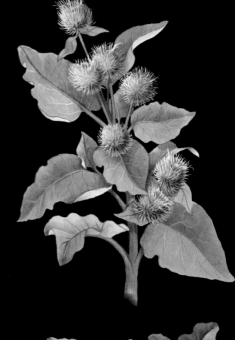

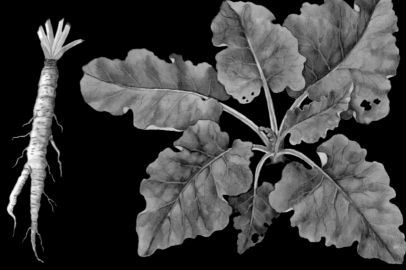

Burdock is another one of those pesky weeds that people hate having on their property, mainly because of its burrs that will attach to just about anything, particularly pet fur. However, it's one of the best detoxifying herbs around and is part of the Essiac formula for treating certain cancers. It grows mainly in waste places, meadows, and woods, and can grow up to 1.8 metres tall. The lower leaves are large, wavy, and heart-shaped, covered with fine hairs, and light grey on the underside. The upper leaves are smaller and oval-shaped with less of the downy covering. The flowerheads are purple and enclosed in a round spiny shell with prickles that hook onto everything that passes by. The long taproot is collected after the first year of growth in early spring, sliced and dried quickly for later use, or eaten fresh as a vegetable. Do not confuse with Rhubarb leaves, which are toxic.

MEDICINAL USES:

Skin diseases, blood purification, urinary and kidney problems, arthritis, PMS

- Contains many minerals, especially iron, that make it valuable for the blood. Beneficial as a detoxifier and blood and liver tonic, as it promotes sweating and detoxifies the epidermal tissues, assists in absorption of nutrients, aids digestion, and relieves bloating and water retention. It works best if used in moderate doses over a long period of time. The seed is said to be better for acute illnesses, whereas the root is more beneficial for chronic problems of the kidneys, bladder, skin, and bowels, and is more permanent.
- Alleviates the pain of arthritis, rheumatism, sciatica, and lumbago by its diuretic action, which increases the removal of urine and toxic substances.
- Due to its ability to increase circulation to the skin and its mucilaginous, demulcent nature it helps chronic skin eruptions like acne, psoriasis, eczema, boils, herpes. It can be taken internally in an infusion and/or used externally as a wash or poultice. Crushed seeds can be poulticed on bruises, the leaves can be applied on burns, ulcers, or sores, on the forehead to relieve headache, or used on the scalp to relieve itchiness or dandruff. Some studies have shown it may even inhibit cancer growth.
- Digestive herb, the bitterness in the leaf stimulates bile production, cleanses the liver and repairs the damaging effects of alcohol; the demulcent quality soothes the digestive tract and contains inulin, which feeds healthy bacteria.
- Eliminates harmful acids from the kidneys, improves filtration, and heals cystitis.
- Regulates the menstrual cycle, relieves symptoms of mastitis and menopause, eases swollen prostate glands.

OTHER USES:
- The stalk, when cut before the flower opens and peeled and boiled, makes a tasty vegetable.
- The young leaves can be eaten fresh in salads, but are slightly laxative.
- The root may be boiled and eaten like carrots.

DECOCTION: Mix 2 tsp. dried root in 2 cups boiling water; soak overnight, boil again in the morning, and simmer 5–10 minutes. Drink 3 times a day.

TINCTURE: Burdock and Red Clover make a good blood tonic. Burdock can be combined with Yellow Dock root or Dandelion root to detoxify and stimulate digestion.

IMPORTANT: When gathering seeds, be careful to remove the splinters clinging to them before use, as they can be extremely irritating.

CALAMUS

Acorus calamus
Acorus americanus

FAMILY: *Acoraceae*

OTHER NAMES: Sweet flag, Sweet sedge, Flagroot, Bitterroot, *Fr.* Acore, Belle-Angelique

PARTS USED: Rhizome (dried)

CHARACTERISTICS: Acrid, slightly warm, aromatic, pungent, bitter

SYSTEMS AFFECTED: Heart, liver, spleen, stomach

ACTIONS: Stimulant, carminative, antispasmodic, antimicrobial, expectorant, emetic, demulcent, mild sedative

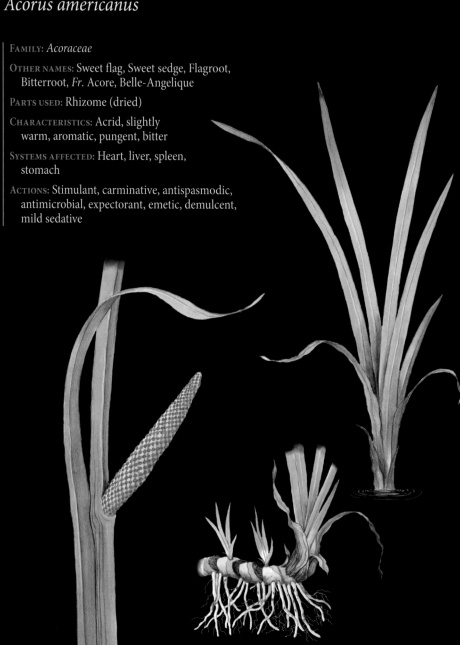

This perennial semi-aquatic plant is found around marshes and lakes and looks very similar to Sweet Flag or Cattail until their flowers come out. Erect, sword-shaped, yellow-green leaves are 0.5–0.9 metres tall, and have a pleasant odour when crushed. The rhizome is buried in mud and is about the thickness of a finger with leaf scars and numerous rootlets. The flower stem arises from the axils of the outer leaves, from one side. Projecting outward at an angle is the actual flower: a cylindrical spike covered with small, greenish-yellow, fragrant flowers. Gather the rhizome in late fall or early spring and dry before using.

MEDICINAL USES:

Digestive discomfort, anxiety, anorexia, lack of mental focus, colds

- With a combination of bitter and aromatic spicy properties, Calamus is a great medicine for deficient, sluggish digestion. Eases hyperacidity in the stomach, flatulence, dyspepsia, colic, heartburn, cramps; stimulates appetite and peristalsis in the stomach; relieves motion sickness and eases anxiety. Just chew a small piece of dried root (about ½ tbsp.)—it's quite bitter, but it works.
- Add to bathwater to calm the nerves, reduce stress, and ease fatigue and anxiety. Chewing the root also helps maintain concentration and focus, eases panic attacks, and enhances awareness.
- The Mi'kmaq consider it to be a sacred plant and often carry the root around to prevent disease or chew on it to relieve indigestion, clear the throat, or increase endurance and concentration. It was also reported to have been used to treat diabetes.
- Its aromatic oils and strong antimicrobial action help ease sore throat, chest colds, stuffy sinuses, laryngitis.
- Enhances libido; relieves pain of endometriosis.

OTHER USES:
- The highly aromatic volatile oil is used for perfumes.
- Can be used as a spice or flavouring for beer or gin.
- Burning dried leaves can be used as a smudge.
- As a strewing herb to keep away insects.

COLD INFUSION: Steep the root in a jar (2 cups) of cold water 10–12 hours; drink throughout the day.

CANDIES: Cut the root into thin slices and boil in syrup, drain and dry in a warm oven, for indigestion. Cut root into thin slices and parboil in water, changing once or twice to reduce the bitterness, then simmer in simple syrup (2 parts sugar, 1 part water), just to cover, until most of the syrup is absorbed. Drain, roll in sugar if desired. Preheat oven to 200°F and bake mixture on a cookie sheet until dry.

IMPORTANT: Do not consume in large doses, as it can cause vomiting. Avoid during pregnancy.

CHICKWEED

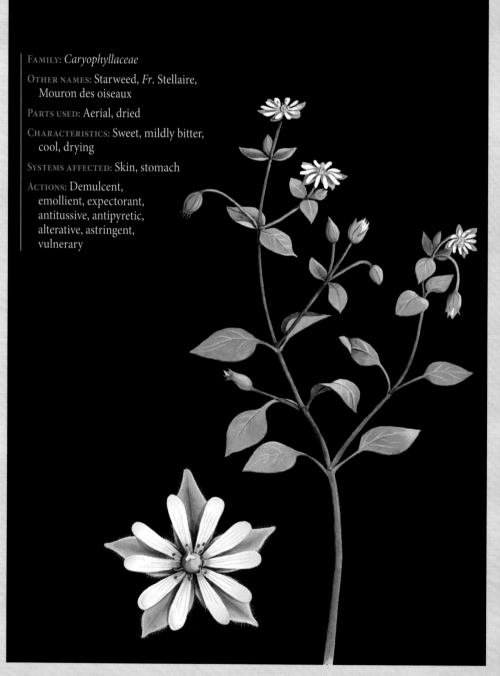

Stellaria media

FAMILY: *Caryophyllaceae*

OTHER NAMES: Starweed, *Fr.* Stellaire, Mouron des oiseaux

PARTS USED: Aerial, dried

CHARACTERISTICS: Sweet, mildly bitter, cool, drying

SYSTEMS AFFECTED: Skin, stomach

ACTIONS: Demulcent, emollient, expectorant, antitussive, antipyretic, alterative, astringent, vulnerary

Chickweed is a small, creeping annual, with weak, many-branched stems up to 40 cm. long that trail along the ground. Its scientific name, *Stellaria media*, means "little stars," which perfectly describes the shape of its flowers. This plant is identified by a line of hairs running up one side of its stem, then continuing along the opposite side when it reaches a pair of leaves. The opposite leaves are succulent, smooth, oval, and pointed. The small white flowers have 5 petals that are deeply divided, making it seem like there are 10 petals, and are only open for 12 hours on fine days. In the rain they droop, and at night the leaves fold over the delicate flowers and protect the tip of the shoot. They begin blooming in early spring and continue through till fall. The seedpod is a small capsule with teeth that, when ripe, shake the seeds when the wind blows. It grows in fields and waste areas and should be collected between May and July.

MEDICINAL USES:

Skin irritations, weight loss, sore throat, fever, inflammation

- Whole plant is edible, nutritious, high in vitamins and minerals, and may be added to a salad or used as a potherb. Contains saponins, which improve absorption of nutrients. Works well as a cleansing herb and spring tonic. Helps with weight loss, and is mildly diuretic and laxative.
- In the form of an ointment or poultice, chickweed has a cooling and drying effect on skin irritations, itches, rashes, wounds, ulcers, boils, eczema, and psoriasis. A fresh poultice will actually heat up as it draws out infection from the body. Its emollient properties make it very soothing. As a decoction it can be used to treat rheumatic pain, wounds, or ulcers. It may also be added to bathwater to soothe inflammation, sunburn, or hemorrhoids.
- Tincture of the fresh herb has been used successfully to dissolve cysts and benign tumors.
- Treats fevers, inflammation, and other hot diseases. Soothes sore throat and lungs, reduces swelling and irritation in the sinuses.

POULTICE: Apply fresh chopped herb directly onto sores or wounds, cover with a clean towel, and leave for up to 3 hours. Replace if poultice begins to feel warm. If using older woody plants, cook in water for several minutes and cool before applying.

INFUSION: Mix ¼ cup fresh herb with 2½ cups boiling water, infuse 10 minutes, strain. Drink throughout the day. Great for people recovering from an illness.

TINCTURE: Fill a jar (any size) with fresh chopped herb, cover with vodka, and let it sit for at least 6 weeks. Use 1 ml. 2–3 times a day for several months.

OIL: Macerate fresh or dried herb in olive oil for 4 days, then squeeze through cheesecloth. Combines well with Yarrow or St. John's Wort oils.

CHICORY

Cichorium intybus

Family: *Asteraceae*

Other names: Blue sailors, Coffeeweed, Succory, *Fr.* Chicorée sauvage

Parts used: Root, leaves

Characteristics: Cooling, slightly bitter

Systems affected: Liver, kidneys, stomach

Actions: Stomachic, antibacterial, antifungal, anthelmintic, tonic, mild diuretic, sedative, mild laxative, anti-inflammatory

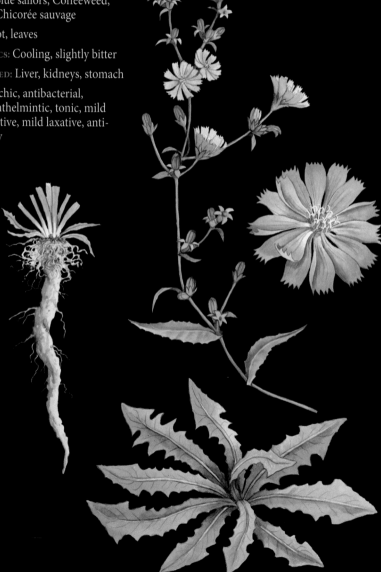

Chicory is a hardy biennial or perennial originating from Europe and Asia, and has a long history of use in these countries as a medicinal plant. It grows almost a metre tall and can be found along roadsides and in fields from early summer right through to the fall. The stems branch out of a hairy rosette similar to the dandelion, and stretch in all directions looking somewhat angular and sparsely clothed with small leaves. Like the dandelion, chicory also oozes a milky sap when cut. The delicate blue–mauve flowers appear in clusters of 2 or 3 and close up early in the afternoon. It has a large taproot, which is woody in the wild but when cultivated is large and fleshy and may be roasted and ground as a coffee substitute.

MEDICINAL USES:

Liver ailments, gallstones, digestive problems, swelling, and inflammation

- Benefits the liver; helps to treat jaundice, gallstones. The root contains inulin, which has little impact on blood sugar, making it suitable for diabetics. The juice of the leaves or a tea made from the flowering plant promote the production of bile and is useful for treating gastritis, flatulence, slow digestion, and chronic constipation. A decoction of the root can be used as a tonic, laxative, or diuretic, and it cools heat, stimulates appetite, and tones the intestines.
- Romans macerated the root in honey wine to alleviate painful urination, jaundice, and kidney stones. Before the wars in Afghanistan, a decoction of the roots was used to fight malaria.
- Some research has been done on its effect on the heart, as it appears to slow a rapid heart rate and may have an antioxidant effect on LDL (bad cholesterol).
- Poultices made from bruised Chicory leaves may reduce swelling, inflammation, and arthritic pain.
- Reduces anxiety and stress; when mixed with coffee it nullifies the effects of caffeine.
- Antibacterial and anti-fungal properties. Decreases biofilm formation and adhesion of bacteria to cells in cases of candida, streptococcus, and other pathogenic organisms.

OTHER USES:
- Root can be roasted and ground up as a coffee substitute.
- Used as feed for animals to remove parasites.
- Young leaves can be eaten fresh in salads; older leaves and stems can be boiled and eaten as a vegetable.

DECOCTION: Put 2 tsp. dried herb or roasted root in 1 cup of water, bring to a boil, and simmer 10–15 minutes. Strain and store in a glass jar. Drink 1–1½ cups per day.

IMPORTANT: Do not use while pregnant or breastfeeding. Use in moderation over a short period of time.

CINQUEFOIL

Potentilla canadensis (Dwarf Cinquefoil)
Potentilla norvegica (Rough Cinquefoil)
Potentilla simplex (Common Cinquefoil)
Potentilla recta (Rough-fruited Cinquefoil)
Potentilla reptans (Creeping Cinquefoil)

FAMILY: *Rosaceae*

PARTS USED: Herb, root

CHARACTERISTICS: Bitter, slightly sweet, cool

SYSTEMS AFFECTED: Upper intestines, stomach, skin

ACTIONS: Astringent (especially the root), febrifuge, anti-inflammatory, disinfectant

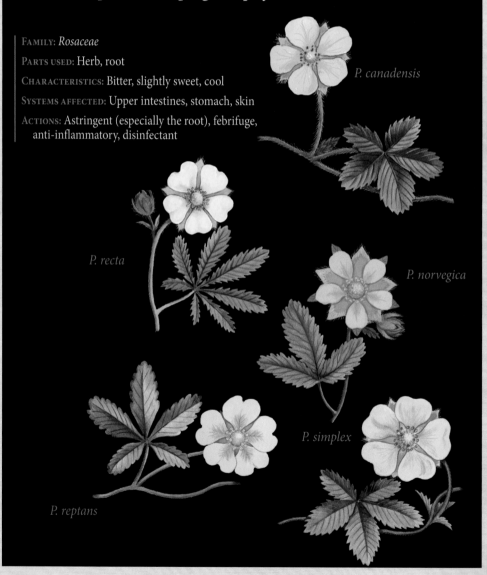

P. canadensis

P. recta

P. norvegica

P. simplex

P. reptans

The Cinquefoil, or "five-leaf," is a small, hairy, native perennial. There are many different species growing in Eastern Canada, all of which are very similar physically as well as medicinally. Leaves are compound divided into 3, 5, or 7 sharply toothed, oblong leaflets. The yellow flowers grow on long leafless stalks out of the axils of the leaves. They have 5 petals and bloom from June to September. The plant creeps along the ground, sending out hairy runners, similar to the Strawberry plant. They may be gathered while in flower—preferably in June—and dried in the shade for later use. The root is best if dug up in April.

MEDICINAL USES:

Inflammation, fever, mouth infections, diarrhea

- Indigenous peoples have used Cinquefoil leaves for centuries to stem bleeding (contains tannic acid).
- Cools intermittent fevers (hot and cold) and inflammation.
- Infusion used as a mouthwash can soothe a toothache, or relieve mouth sores, bleeding gums, or infections. Juice or decoction mixed with honey can be used to treat hoarseness or cough.
- General disinfectant and astringent to stop bleeding or soothe burns.
- Root boiled in apple cider vinegar can relieve pain from sores, shingles, or inflammation.
- Relieves stomach ulcers, inflammation in the upper digestive tract, and diarrhea.
- Young leaves are good in salads.

FOLKLORE: This plant has been used for centuries as protection from witches and sorcery and was often hung over doors or windows to prevent disturbances. Images of the flower were carved into churches dating from the eleventh century. It was a symbol of strength and honour; the leaf was emblazoned on the shields of medieval knights to signify the five senses, or the power of self-mastery. Lovers used it in love potions and fishers added it to their nets to increase catches.

INFUSION: 1–2 tsp. herb in 1 cup boiling water, infuse 10–15 minutes. Drink 2–3 times a day.

IMPORTANT: Not recommended for use during pregnancy.

COLTSFOOT

Tussilago farfara

FAMILY: *Asteraceae*

OTHER NAMES: Horsehoof, Coughwort, Son-before-the-father, *Fr.* Pas d'âne

PARTS USED: Dried leaves and flowers

CHARACTERISTICS: Bitter, sweet, neutral

SYSTEMS AFFECTED: Lungs

ACTIONS: Antitussive, expectorant, demulcent, anti-inflammatory, astringent, diuretic, emollient

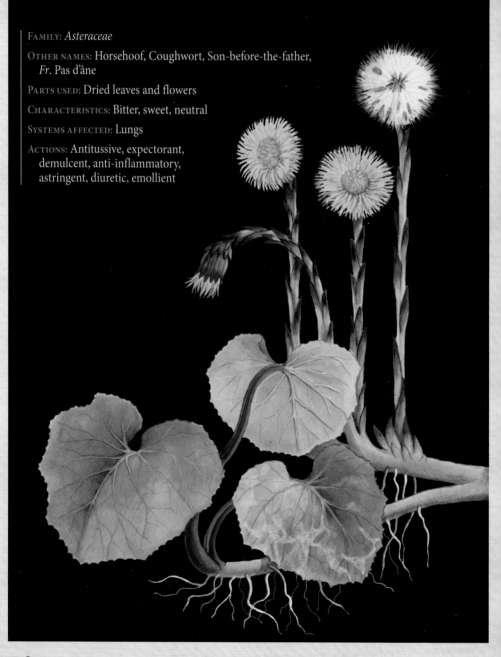

Native to Europe, Coltsfoot (or Tussilago, which means "cough dispeller") is one of the first wildflowers to bloom in early spring, but its leaves don't appear until long after the flowers have opened. The bright yellow flowers open in sunshine and close in cloudy weather, and are often mistaken for Dandelions. The difference is Coltsfoot's stem, which is covered in brown-tipped scales and grows upward from a creeping rhizome to 7.5–30 cm. tall. Rosettes of the stalked leaves usually grow in after the flower has gone to seed. Each rosette is the shape of a horse's hoof, has irregular toothed edges, and is covered with a woolly coating, which becomes smooth and waxy on top as the leaf matures, with a grey woolly underside. The soft seed heads resemble those of the Dandelion and are used by birds to line their nests. Coltsfoot typically grows along cliffs, ditches, or riverbanks and tolerates wet areas. Flowers should be gathered before fully bloomed and dried in the shade; leaves should be harvested in early summer, and chopped and dried for later use.

MEDICINAL USES:

Lung complaints, coughs

- Contains mucilage, which soothes mucous membranes and is useful for upper respiratory problems with a dry, unproductive cough that is chronic and persistent, as well as asthma. When fresh, the herb can be used in teas; it has a liquorice-like flavour. It is also used dried in infusions, syrups, and cough drops, or it can be smoked.
- Crushed fresh leaves can be applied to burns and skin ailments, boils, insect bites, abscesses, or inflamed areas.
- Indigenous peoples and colonists once soaked blankets in hot infusion to wrap around a patient with whooping cough.
- Mild diuretic for cystitis.
- Basis of British Herb Tobacco which also contains Buckbean, Eyebright, Betony, Rosemary, Thyme, Lavender, and Chamomile.

OTHER USES: Young leaves may be used fresh in salads or sautéed as a vegetable. Seed heads were once used as mattress stuffing.

INFUSION: Mix 2 tbsp. dried herb in 2 cups of boiling water. Keep warm in a Thermos beside the bed to soothe morning coughs. Add honey and Anise or Fennel seed if desired. Also works well with Mullein, Thyme, and Liquorice.

IMPORTANT: Contains pyrrolizidine alkaloids, which may harm the liver, although some are destroyed during the decoction process. Do not consume in large doses or over a period of more than 2 weeks. Should not be given to small children. Avoid use during pregnancy.

DANDELION

Taraxacum officinale

FAMILY: *Asteraceae*

OTHER NAMES: *Fr.* Pissenlit, Dent-de-lion

PARTS USED: Roots, leaves, flowers

CHARACTERISTICS: Leaves: cool, bitter, drying. Roots: sweet, bitter, cool

SYSTEMS AFFECTED: Liver, spleen, stomach, kidney, bladder

ACTIONS: Diuretic (especially roots), tonic, alterative, cholagogue, laxative

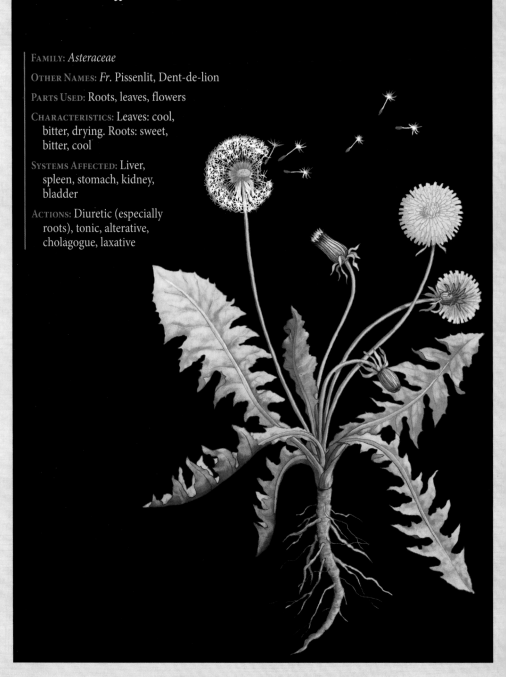

Although it has been considered a pesky weed ever since well-groomed lawns became popular, the Dandelion remains one of the most effective (and widely available) medicinal herbs. Easily identified on every lawn and field early in the spring, it is a hardy perennial with a basal rosette of deeply toothed leaves above a central taproot. There are several slender, hollow stalks emerging from each rosette, which contain a milky latex. All stalks are leafless with one composite yellow flowerhead, which opens in the morning and closes up when the sun goes down. These flowers mature into white fluffy spheres, which are actually seeds with tiny hairy parachutes to help disperse them easily in the wind. Harvest the leaves in spring when they are tender; roots can be harvested in fall, and should be split longitudinally and dried for later use.

MEDICINAL USES:

Kidney and liver disorders, urinary tract infections, skin eruptions, stomach pains

- As a general cleanser, it stimulates and tonifies, aids bile production and digestion, balances digestive enzymes, and encourages the elimination of toxins from the body. It clears liver congestion, and helps in the treatment of jaundice, cirrhosis, and enlargement of the liver.
- High in mineral content, it makes a great spring tonic, and is a rich source of vitamins A and C, potassium, and calcium.
- A strong decoction of Dandelion root is useful in clearing obstructions from the spleen, pancreas, bladder, and kidneys.
- A powerful diuretic (especially the leaves), it decreases high blood pressure and edema without depleting the body of potassium, the way many pharmaceuticals do.
- Treats anemia with many nutritive minerals; purifies the blood.
- Combined with Endive and Chicory, the young leaves make a great cleansing salad and promote regularity.
- Root tea, taken 4–6 times a day, combined with a light diet of broths, rice, and mung beans can benefit those with hepatitis by reducing inflammation.
- Clears acne and other inflammatory skin conditions, especially if combined with Burdock root. Also, the latex can be rubbed on the skin to remove warts.

OTHER USES:
- The flowers can be made into wine or jelly or added to salads.
- The roasted root makes a nice hot beverage.

DECOCTION: Combine 2–3 tsp. thinly sliced root with 1 cup of water. Bring to a boil and simmer 10–15 minutes. Cool, sweeten with honey if desired. Drink 3 times a day. May be combined with Burdock root.

TINCTURE: 1 tsp. per day.

IMPORTANT: Do not use Dandelions from lawns that have been treated with chemicals.

ELDER

Sambucus canadensis

FAMILY: *Caprifoliaceae*

OTHER NAMES: Common elder, Black elder, Pipe tree, *Fr.* Sureau blanc

PARTS USED: Flowers, berries, leaves

CHARACTERISTICS: Flowers: Sweet, cool, drying. Berries and leaves: Acrid, bitter, cool.

SYSTEMS AFFECTED: Lungs, liver

ACTIONS: Flowers: Diaphoretic, anti-catarrhal, mildly sedative. Berries: Diaphoretic, diuretic, laxative, antioxidant. Leaves: emollient, vulnerary, purgative, expectorant, diuretic

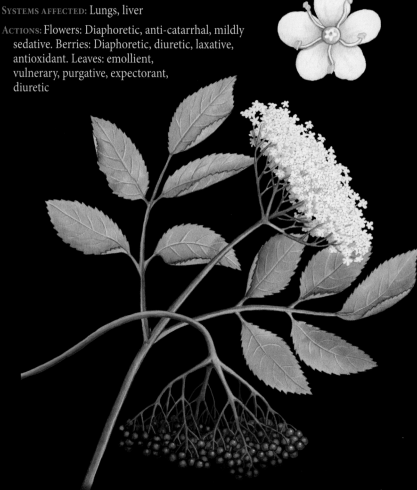

Sambucus canadensis is an indigenous shrub that very closely resembles its European relative, *Sambucus nigra*, both in appearance and medicinal properties. It grows to a height of 1.5–3.5 metres, with paired opposite leaves and one extra at the end of each branch, each finely serrated, oval, and pointed. The whitish flowers appear in July growing in many large umbels and having a somewhat peculiar aroma. They develop into berries in the fall, first a greenish colour and eventually turning to black. They should only be used when completely ripe. Do not confuse with the Red Elder berry, which is poisonous. The young branches contain a soft pith that is easily removed and was once used to make pipes or musical instruments; however, the fresh stems are poisonous and should be aged at least a year. Flowers should be harvested gently, removed from their stalks, and dried quickly in a cool oven. The berries may be gathered in the fall and dried or frozen for later use. They should not be consumed raw. Store in an airtight container.

MEDICINAL USES:

Colds, flu, sinusitis, skin ailments

- Berries are nutritious, rich in antioxidants, flavonoids, vitamins, and minerals.
- In first stages of cold or flu, upper respiratory tract infection, sinusitis, hay fever, Elder flower tea promotes expectoration and perspiration and can be taken hot before going to bed. It can be mixed with Peppermint if desired. Syrup of the berries (below) has been proven to reduce symptoms and duration of colds and flu if taken at the first sign.
- Flowers and leaves are used in ointments and lotions to treat burns, rashes, bruises, sprains, minor skin ailments, and to diminish wrinkles.
- Tea made from the flowers is a mild laxative and diuretic and warm compresses may reduce pain of rheumatism, arthritis, and inflamed swellings. A cold infusion is said to be effective in relief of swollen glands.
- Strained Elder flower tea that has been cooled with ¼ tsp. salt added per cup makes a good eyewash to reduce inflammation.
- Elder berry wine was once used to ease pain associated with arthritis.

FOLKLORE: There are many myths surrounding this bush that date far back and span across many cultures. Medieval beliefs held it to be a symbol of death and bad luck. In Scandinavia it was believed a dryad, Hyldemoer, lived in an Elder tree, and if it was cut or used for furniture she would forever haunt those responsible. In England in the seventeenth century it was thought that the tree would provide protection against witches, and people often carried a twig in their pockets to prevent rheumatism.

INFUSION FOR FLU WITH FEVER: Mix equal parts Elder flower, Yarrow, and Peppermint to make 2 tbsp. in 1 cup of boiling water (3 or 4 slices of fresh Ginger root may also be added). Take a warm bath and drink hot before bed.

SYRUP: Place 1⅓ cup frozen or 1 cup dried Elder berries in a pot, add enough water to cover. Add 1 tsp. Cinnamon, ½ tsp. Cloves, and a few slices of fresh Ginger, and simmer over low heat, stirring and mashing until mixture is mushy and reduced by half. Strain liquid into a measuring cup, and add an equal amount of honey to the juice. Add a squirt of lemon juice and/or brandy if desired (helps to preserve it). Ratio should be 20:80 alcohol to syrup. Store in a jar in the fridge, take 1 tbsp. every hour at the onset of cold or flu, then 3–4 times a day.

IMPORTANT: Do not confuse with Red Elder berry (*S. racemosa*) as it is poisonous. Fresh roots, leaves, stems, and raw berries are toxic and should not be consumed.

EVENING PRIMROSE

Oenothera biennis

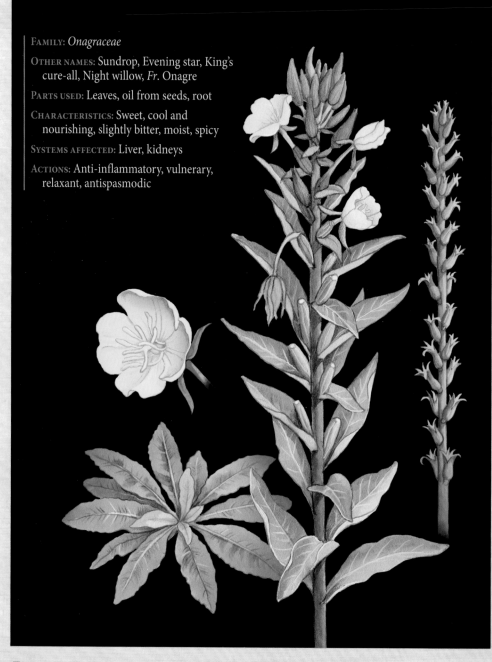

FAMILY: *Onagraceae*

OTHER NAMES: Sundrop, Evening star, King's cure-all, Night willow, *Fr.* Onagre

PARTS USED: Leaves, oil from seeds, root

CHARACTERISTICS: Sweet, cool and nourishing, slightly bitter, moist, spicy

SYSTEMS AFFECTED: Liver, kidneys

ACTIONS: Anti-inflammatory, vulnerary, relaxant, antispasmodic

Evening Primrose has a long history in North America, both for its medicinal proper-ties and its use as a vegetable. The entire plant is edible and was a nutritious source of food for pre-contact Indigenous peoples, particularly the boiled root, which has a peppery taste. An erect biennial, it forms a rosette of basal leaves in the first year. In its second year, the hairy stems arise from the centre to a height of 0.9–1.2 metres, bearing yellow, delicately fragrant flowers all along the stalks, with new ones forming until late in the fall. They are replaced by hairy green seed pods that open into four sections to spread their seeds. The common name derives from the flowers, which only open in the evening early in the season to accommodate the flying insects that pollinate them. The root is best when harvested in the plant's first year. The seeds, the most active part medicinally, are gathered when the pods mature late in the summer. The early leaves as well as the flowers can be eaten in salads, or leaves can be cooked and eaten as greens.

MEDICINAL USES:

Hypertension, anxiety, PMS, arthritis, eczema

- Seed oil: contains gamma-linolenic acid (GLA), an unsaturated fatty acid, which plays a role in brain function, skin and hair growth, bone health, and regulates the hormones and repro-ductive system. It also helps eczema and asthma due to allergies, and relieves inflammation and acne.
- The seed oil may also be used as a muscle relaxant to calm nerves and irritation, anxiety, chronic headaches, PMS, menstrual cramps, breast tenderness, and symptoms of menopause. Some studies have shown GLA may increase fertility.
- Anti-clotting, the seed oil is useful in treating hypertension and preventing heart attacks caused by thrombosis or blood clots; reduces blood pressure. It also helps relieve the pain of rheumatoid arthritis and diabetic neuropathy. May lessen inflammation and damage caused by multiple sclerosis.
- Leaves and mashed root can be eaten or used as a poultice for healing wounds, bruises, boils, swelling, hemorrhoids, redness, and irritation.

COUGH SYRUP: Ground dried root may be mixed with warm honey for an effective cough syrup; take as needed.

EYEBRIGHT

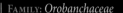

Euphrasia nemorosa

FAMILY: *Orobanchaceae*

OTHER NAMES: Meadow Eyebright, *Fr.* Euphraise, Casse-lunette

PARTS USED: Aerial, dried

CHARACTERISTICS: Bitter, mildly astringent, cool

SYSTEMS AFFECTED: Liver, lungs

ACTIONS: Astringent, anti-inflammatory, expectorant, anti-catarrhal, tonic

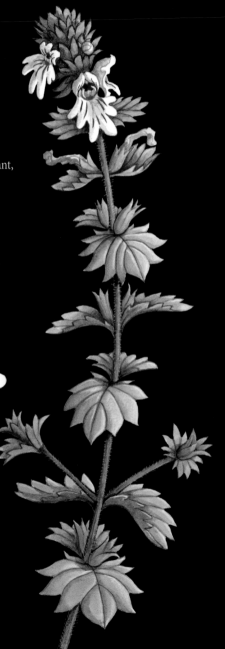

This small, delicate annual has been used for centuries to treat eye diseases. Growing up to 20 cm. high, it has square, downy, branching stems with notched leaves that grow in opposite pairs. The tiny white flowers have purplish and yellow markings inside, which herbalists claim resemble a bloodshot eye. There are two lips: the lower one has 3 lobes; the upper one has 2 that arch over the stamens. Eyebright is semi-parasitic, getting part of its nourishment from surrounding grasses, to which it attaches underground suckers. It is best collected in July and August when the flowers are in bloom; cut just above the root.

MEDICINAL USES:

Eye diseases, throat irritations, eczema

- Treats various diseases of the eye, such as pink eye, conjunctivitis, red or irritated eyes, or styes, and can be taken internally and/or externally (should be sterile if applied directly to the eye). Contains vitamins A, B, C, and E, which are known to improve eye health. Increases elasticity in the optic tissues.
- Tea made from leaves, stems, and flowers used to treat symptoms of sinus congestion, allergies, and colds, particularly if the discharge is thin and watery. Relieves inflammation of the mucous membranes.
- Poultice can soothe eczema, acne, and wounds.

INFUSION: Steep 1 tsp. of dried herb in 1 cup of boiling water. Infuse 5 to 10 minutes. Drink 3 times a day.

TINCTURE: 6–12 drops, 3 times a day.

EYEWASH: Allow infusion to cool, then strain. Use a sterile eyecup to rinse eyes. Use within 24 hours.

- ALTERNATIVELY: Pour 2 tbsp. freshly boiled water over 10 drops of tincture. Cool just to lukewarm, fill a sterilized eyecup about a third full and rinse eye in solution. Discard used solution and repeat for other eye.

COMPRESS: Mix 1 tsp. dried herb in 2 cups of water, boil 10 minutes, let cool until lukewarm. Moisten a sterile cloth in liquid, wring slightly, and place over eyes for 15 minutes.

IMPORTANT: Do not use if you have had eye surgery or wear contact lenses. Test for allergies before using on the eyes.

FEVERFEW

Tanacetum (Chrysanthemum) parthenium

FAMILY: *Asteraceae*

OTHER NAMES: Featherfew, Featherfoil, Flintwort, Bachelor's buttons, *Fr.* Grande camomille

PARTS USED: Aerial

CHARACTERISTICS: Aromatic, bitter

SYSTEMS AFFECTED: Intestines, stomach

ACTIONS: Febrifuge, anti-inflammatory, emmenagogue, tonic, analgesic, aperient, carminative, vermifuge

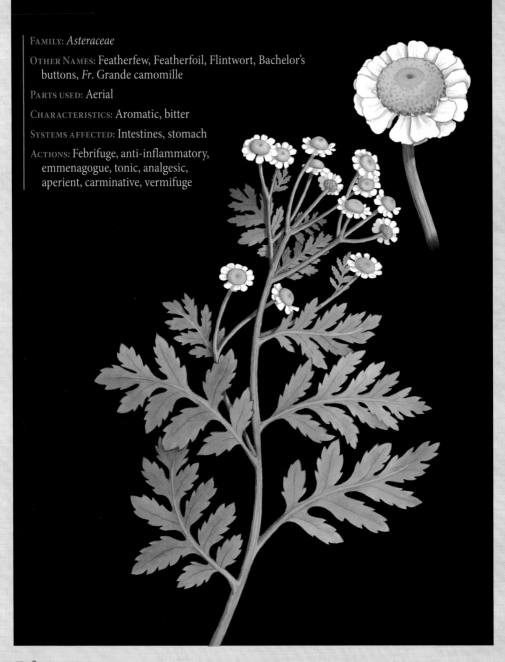

This erect perennial or biennial is a European native that is now common throughout North America but grows mostly in gardens, occasionally escaping into the wild or surviving near old homesteads. Its branched leafy stem is furrowed, about half a metre high, with alternate pinnate leaves, its leaflets gashed and toothed. The compound flowers resemble a small daisy, its center convex and bright yellow, the petals often doubled. It flowers throughout the summer and is aromatic; bees dislike it and will keep their distance. Gather in early summer; as it is best used fresh, it is preferable to freeze for later use.

MEDICINAL USES:

Migraines, fevers, irregular menstruation, stomach upset, arthritis

- As its name suggests, Feverfew was once known for its fever-reducing properties and usefulness for treating the common cold; however, there are other herbs that have proven more effective such as Elder berry, Yarrow, and Boneset. Its main use now is in preventing and treating migraines. In several double-blind, placebo-controlled studies where migraine patients took capsules of Feverfew every day, they reported less-intense migraines and related symptoms after 12 weeks. Like many herbs, a small and regular dose over a long period of time works better than taking a large amount over a short period of time.
- Increases appetite, improves digestion, helps relieve colic and colitis.
- May help reduce skin inflammation and relieve dermatitis.
- Uterine stimulant, it promotes menstruation, eases irregularities and cramps. Tones the womb after childbirth.
- There is some promising research into using Feverfew and St. John's Wort for diabetic peripheral neuropathy.
- May relieve the pain and inflammation of arthritis and rheumatism.
- Some claim it will relieve tinnitus and Ménière's disease.

FOLKLORE: Planted around one's dwelling, it was said to purify the air and prevent disease. Often used to ward off insects.

INFUSION: 1–2 tsp. fresh herb to 1 cup of boiling water; cool. Drink ½ cup, 2 times a day.

TINCTURE: 6–12 drops, 3 times a day.

IMPORTANT: Not recommended if pregnant or breastfeeding. Avoid if you are prone to allergies. If taking for more than 1 week and wish to stop, take care to reduce dosage gradually, as stopping all at once may cause headaches, anxiety, muscle stiffness, and joint pain. May increase the risk of bleeding; avoid if you are on blood thinners. Ask your doctor before taking if you are on any medications. Do not give to children under 2 years of age.

FIREWEED

Chamaenerion (Epilobium) angustifolium

FAMILY: *Onagraceae*

OTHER NAMES: Willow herb, Purple firetop, Blooming Sally, *Fr.* Épilobe, Herbe-à-feu

PARTS USED: Roots, leaves, flowers

CHARACTERISTICS: Sweet, cool, drying

SYSTEMS AFFECTED: Lungs, digestive tract, reproductive organs

ACTIONS: Antispasmodic, antiseptic, demulcent, astringent, anti-inflammatory, emollient, laxative, anthelmintic

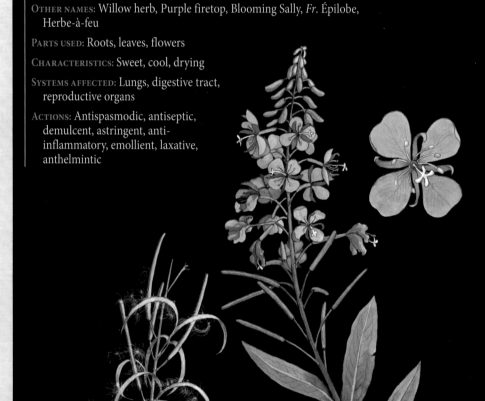

This colourful flower is noted for being one of the first plants to appear after a wildfire, for it thrives on burnt or disturbed land and can become invasive very quickly as it spreads both by self-seeding and rhizomes. Native to North America, it is a perennial herb growing up to 1.8 metres tall, with magenta flowers that bloom from July through to September. They bloom low on the stem at first, and throughout the summer they work their way up to the top. In the fall, the seed pods split open and the plant tops become white and feathery, the tufts of white hair distributing the seeds on the wind. The willow-like alternate leaves are dark green above and silvery underneath, with a lighter central vein. The lateral veins are unique; they don't extend to the outer edge but loop together near the margin. Young shoots may be harvested in the spring and eaten fresh in salads. Leaves can be picked early in the summer and dried in a paper bag, then stored in a glass jar for later use. The root should be dug in the fall and may be used fresh, and mashed as a poultice to soothe inflammation.

MEDICINAL USES:

Asthma, coughs, irritable bowel, skin problems

- The whole plant is edible and is a gentle but effective anti-inflammatory. Rich in vitamin C, calcium, and iron.
- Antispasmodic, demulcent, and high in mucilage, it soothes mucus membranes, and a cool decoction of the whole plant can be used to treat whooping cough, asthma, and hiccups.
- Leaf decoctions are anti-inflammatory and good for the stomach and the digestive tract, and soothe and rebalance irritable bowels and diarrhea. Young flowerheads may be infused in oil for treating hemorrhoids.
- Indigenous peoples use the peeled root in poultices for boils or abscesses, or the leaves in compresses for burns, psoriasis, eczema, acne, and wounds. A tea can be made from the whole plant to treat digestive and bronchial problems and internal parasites..
- Current research shows the rhizome, which contains flavonoids and the tannin oenethein B, may be useful in treating benign prostatic hyperplasia (BPH) and possibly prostate cancer.

OTHER USES:
- Young shoots and flowers are good in salads or as a potherb.
- Dried leaves make a nice tea.
- Yields a delicious honey.
- Cordage made from fibrous stems.
- Cottony seed hairs can be used as stuffing or tinder.

INFUSION: Mix 1–2 tsp. dried herb in 1 cup of boiling water. Drink as needed.

GOAT'S BEARD

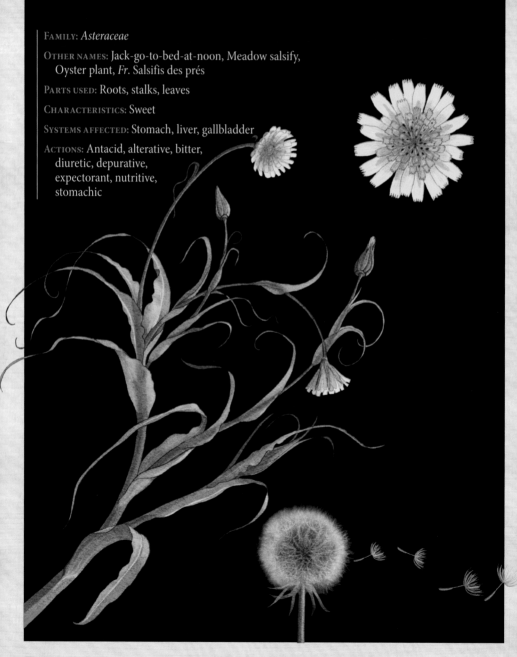

Tragopogon pratensis

FAMILY: *Asteraceae*

OTHER NAMES: Jack-go-to-bed-at-noon, Meadow salsify, Oyster plant, *Fr.* Salsifis des prés

PARTS USED: Roots, stalks, leaves

CHARACTERISTICS: Sweet

SYSTEMS AFFECTED: Stomach, liver, gallbladder

ACTIONS: Antacid, alterative, bitter, diuretic, depurative, expectorant, nutritive, stomachic

Goat's Beard is a biennial herb that was introduced to North America from Europe. It probably got its name from its fluffy grey seed ball—which looks similar to a Dandelion's, but larger—that appears when the flowers have faded. In fact, it is often confused with the Dandelion since its yellow flowers are similar as well; however, the plant itself is much different. Often growing up to 76 cm. tall, it has long, narrow, grass-like leaves, broader at the base, with a tendency to curl at the tips. The yellow flower opens in the morning but closes up before noon, hence the name "Jack-go-to-bed-at-noon." It can be found in fields and along roadsides. The leaves and stems are best harvested in the spring before flowers appear; the long taproot may be collected in the fall.

MEDICINAL USES:

Heartburn, loss of appetite, coughs

- Useful remedy for the liver and gallbladder. Decoction of the roots detoxifies, relieves heartburn, eases stomach upset, and stimulates appetite. Good for diabetics, as it contains inulin and does not raise blood sugar levels.
- Mostly used as a vegetable, the young greens can be eaten fresh in salads, and the stems may be boiled and eaten like asparagus. The roots should be cleaned well, peeled, and sliced, then boiled for about 30 minutes. They can be served like parsnips with butter, or added to stews and soups.
- Syrup made from the root relieves stubborn coughs and bronchitis.
- Was once used as a diuretic and to treat kidney stones, but there are other herbs used now that are more effective.
- An infusion of the flowers may be used in lotions to clear the skin and lighten freckles.

OTHER USES: The milky latex in the stems can be dried and used as chewing gum.

GOLDENROD

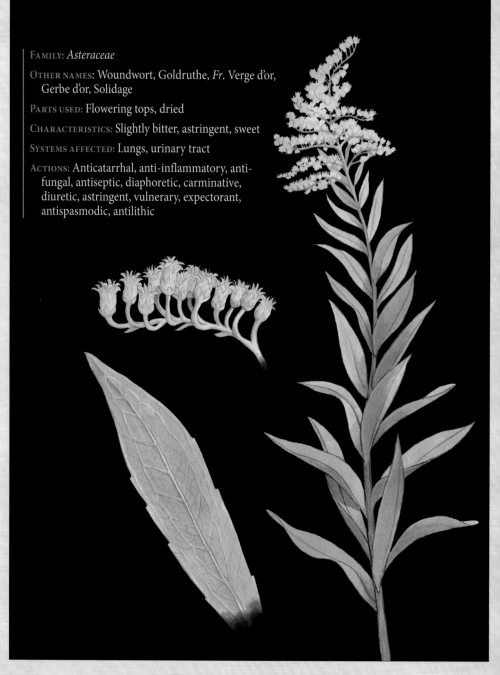

Solidago canadensis

FAMILY: *Asteraceae*

OTHER NAMES: Woundwort, Goldruthe, *Fr.* Verge d'or, Gerbe d'or, Solidage

PARTS USED: Flowering tops, dried

CHARACTERISTICS: Slightly bitter, astringent, sweet

SYSTEMS AFFECTED: Lungs, urinary tract

ACTIONS: Anticatarrhal, anti-inflammatory, anti-fungal, antiseptic, diaphoretic, carminative, diuretic, astringent, vulnerary, expectorant, antispasmodic, antilithic

Solidago, meaning, "to make whole," refers to Goldenrod's ability to restore the body to health and wholeness. Several varieties of Goldenrod grow in Atlantic Canada, *S. canadensis* being one of the native species, which has been used for centuries by Indigenous peoples to heal wounds. Goldenrod grows in many different habitats depending on the species; some prefer dry fields, others wetlands or marshes. It is a perennial with erect, often downy, stems, which branch at the top. The leaves are alternate, elliptical, toothed, and stalked, and the upper ones are smaller than those at the base. The small yellow flowers grow in clusters; the European variety, *S. virgaurea*, has blooms all around the stem, and the Canadian variety, *S. canadensis*, on only one side. Goldenrod should be harvested during flowering—but before the plant is in full bloom—and then dried in the shade.

MEDICINAL USES:

Urinary tract infections and stones, upper respiratory problems, sore throat, skin inflammation, stomach upset, candida

- Astringent, diuretic, and anti-inflammatory, it is useful in the treatment of urinary tract infections, kidney inflammation (nephritis), and helps dissolve kidney stones and gallstones. Combines well with Elder flowers.
- An effective expectorant, it expels mucus and works on the upper respiratory system, soothing coughs, acute or chronic bronchitis, and asthma. Combines well with Thyme for sinus congestion and Mullein for chest infections.
- A good source of rutin, a powerful flavonoid that increases the strength of capillaries and improves the tone of the cardiovascular system.
- Infusion may be used as a gargle to treat sore throat or laryngitis.
- Used for centuries as a wound herb, it is effective in poultices, ointments, and baths for treating slow-healing wounds, burns, eczema, and varicose veins.
- Soothes upset stomach, flatulence, and colic.
- Tincture may be used to desensitize from seasonal allergens like Ragweed.
- Prevents and treats urogenital disorders like yeast infections; infusion may be drunk as a tea or used as a douche.

OTHER USES: Flowers produce a strong yellow dye.

INFUSION: 1 tbsp. fresh or 2–3 tsp. dried herb in 1 cup boiling water 10–15 minutes. Mint or honey may also be added. Drink 3 times a day. May increase urination or coughing/sneezing when you first start using it.

GOLDTHREAD

Coptis trifolia
C. groenlandica

FAMILY: *Ranunculaceae*

OTHER NAMES: Golden root, Canker root, *Fr.* Savoyane, Sabouillane, Coptide du Groenland

PARTS USED: Dried rhizome, roots, stems, leaves

CHARACTERISTICS: Bitter

SYSTEMS AFFECTED: Liver

ACTIONS: Bitter tonic, antibacterial, stomachic, anti-inflammatory

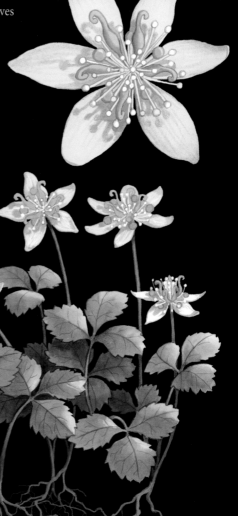

Goldthread is a tiny native perennial herb that has been over-picked to the point where it is now difficult to find. The roots look like a tangled mass of gold thread, and the leaves are evergreen and shiny, somewhat resembling wild Strawberry leaves with 3 leaflets and slightly scalloped edges. The flowers bloom from May to August; a single flower atop a long stem of 7.5–15 cm., with 5–7 delicate white petals. It is found in damp shaded woods, but keep in mind that it is endangered, and unless it is found in abundance, it should be left where it is.

MEDICINAL USES:

Mouth sores, digestive disorders, wounds

- Indigenous peoples have been chewing fresh Goldthread root for centuries to cure mouth sores and thrush; works also for trench mouth and topically for herpes.
- In a sitz bath for rectal fissures or vaginitis, and topically for skin ulcers in general.
- Contains a strong, bitter alkaloid called berberine, which acts as an antibacterial and blood purifier. Good for indigestion and other digestive disorders, jaundice, and general recovery from illness.
- When used with Goldenseal, is said to be effective in helping to destroy one's appetite for alcohol.
- Some studies claim it may be promising in treating HIV, infectious hepatitis, some strains of flu, and even cancer.
- Some Mi'kmaq use Goldthread to treat external sores and wounds by boiling it with sheep fat to make a salve.

DECOCTION: 1 tbsp. fresh finely chopped root (or 1 tsp. dried), add 1 cup of water and boil for 20 minutes. Cool and use as a gargle for mouth sores, or drink 1 tbsp. 3–6 times a day for chronic stomach and digestive inflammation.

TINCTURE: Finely chop entire plant and place in a jar. Cover with 100-proof vodka. Put on lid and leave for 6 weeks, shaking daily. Strain. Drink 1 ml. in a bit of water 3 times a day.

IMPORTANT: Not recommended during pregnancy.

GROUND IVY

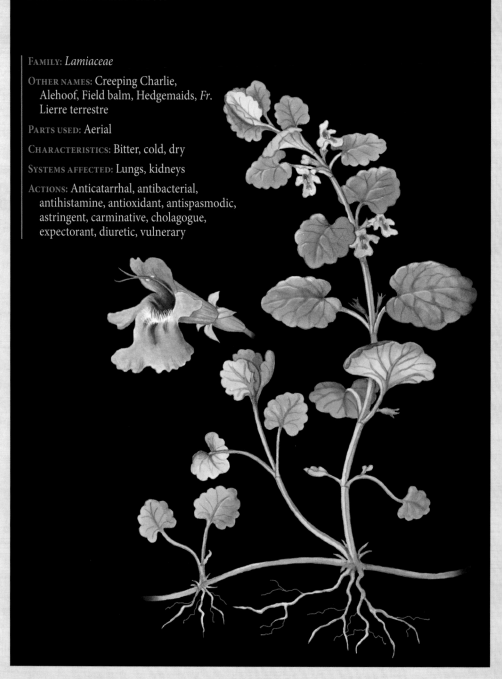

Glechoma hederacea

FAMILY: *Lamiaceae*

OTHER NAMES: Creeping Charlie, Alehoof, Field balm, Hedgemaids, *Fr.* Lierre terrestre

PARTS USED: Aerial

CHARACTERISTICS: Bitter, cold, dry

SYSTEMS AFFECTED: Lungs, kidneys

ACTIONS: Anticatarrhal, antibacterial, antihistamine, antioxidant, antispasmodic, astringent, carminative, cholagogue, expectorant, diuretic, vulnerary

Gardeners have cursed this tenacious little weed relentlessly over the years, but if you search into its history you will discover herbalists once held it in high esteem for its ability to relieve sciatica and skin irritations. Originating in Europe, it is a perennial ground creeper that forms a thick mat and literally takes over lawns and fields. Its leaves are kidney-shaped, stalked, and somewhat downy, with rounded indentations. The tiny flowers are purplish, two-lipped, and grow in clusters. Stems are square, downy, and trailing. It continues to bloom throughout the summer and fall, and the leaves remain green even through the winter. The plant has a balsamic smell due to oil glands on the underside of the leaves. The early Saxons used it to clarify beer before the advent of hops, giving it the name Alehoof. It is best gathered in late May to mid-June when the flowers are fresh. Harvest only the top 50% of the plant, and only from clean areas.

MEDICINAL USES:

Upper respiratory infections, digestive problems, mouth infections, kidney stones

- High in vitamin C, its expectorant properties help to treat damp coughs with fever and it aids in clearing up mucous and phlegm in sinus and ear infections. It is usually combined with other herbs in formulas. Works best in long-term treatment of chronic lung conditions.
- Fresh juice or tea soothes digestive tract in cases of gastritis, enteritis, diarrhea, intestinal gas, colic, and hemorrhoids. May be beneficial to the liver and for removing kidney stones.
- Infusion used as a gargle for mouth infections, gingivitis, sore throat. Especially effective for receding gums and after dental surgery.
- Eases the pain of sciatica, gout, and arthritis; can be added to bathwater to soften skin and ease backaches.
- Poultice soothes the irritation from Nettle stings. Used in combination with Yarrow and Chamomile for sores and abscesses.

FOLKLORE: Tea was believed to be effective for overcoming shyness. Strewing the leaves over the floor is said to create good dreams and peaceful sleep. A garland of Ground Ivy was often worn during the Gaelic pagan festival of Beltane held on May 1 to celebrate the return of the spring flowers.

TINCTURE: Remove leaves from the stems and pack loosely into a sterile Mason jar. Fill with vodka, leaving a few centimetres at the top. Make sure all the leaves are submerged and there is no air trapped between the leaves. Screw on lid and keep in a cupboard 4–6 weeks, shaking often. Strain through cheesecloth and store in an amber dropper bottle. Take 5–10 drops in a glass of water up to 4 times a day.

INFUSION: Steep 2 tsp. fresh (or 1 tsp. dried) herb in 1 cup of boiling water for 10 minutes. Flavour with honey or Peppermint leaves, as it is quite bitter. Makes a nice spring tonic.

IMPORTANT: Not recommended during pregnancy or breastfeeding. Avoid if taking anti-convulsants, sedatives, or mood-altering drugs. May cause throat irritation.

HEAL-ALL

Prunella vulgaris

FAMILY: *Lamiaceae*

OTHER NAMES: Self-heal, All-heal, Prunella, Woundwort, Carpenter weed, *Fr.* Brunelle, Herbe au charpentier, Prunelle commune

PARTS USED: Aerial

CHARACTERISTICS: Slightly bitter, pungent, cold, moistening

SYSTEMS AFFECTED: Liver

ACTIONS: Astringent, vulnerary, tonic, anti-inflammatory, diuretic, haemostatic, antiseptic, antibacterial, antioxidant, antiviral, demulcent

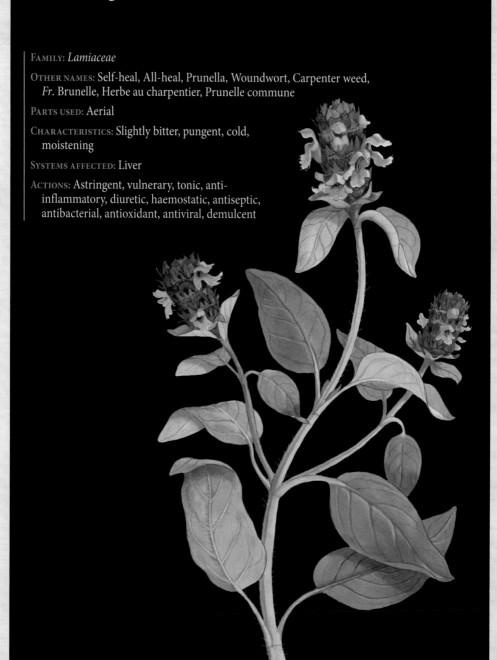

Although this native perennial herb of the Mint family was once used—as its name suggests—to heal just about anything, it has somewhat lost its popularity with herbalists over the years, but new research suggests it could still prove useful. It grows up to 30 cm. high, and is easily identified by its dense cluster of purple flowers at the top of a square stem. They grow in rings around the fat cylindrical spike, looking somewhat ragged since they're never all in bloom at once. Each tubular flower is composed of a 2-lipped calyx with dark red tips, and a 2-lipped purple corolla resembling a throat. Below the flower spike is a set of 2 stalkless leaves, and then more paired opposite leaves on stems branching off of a creeping stem, which sends roots into the soil at intervals. It grows in fields and waste places, and can be picked in the fall and dried for later use.

MEDICINAL USES:

Wounds, sore throat, swollen lymph nodes

- High in antioxidants and antiseptic, a lukewarm infusion makes a nourishing drink; mixed with honey, can be used as a gargle to treat sore throat and mouth infections. Enhances the immune system, and works well with the lymphatic system to reduce swelling, as in mumps, swollen glands, and mastitis. Weak infusion may be used in a sterile eyewash for dry, painful eyes or conjunctivitis.
- Before the Second World War, Heal-all was used extensively to clean wounds and stop hemorrhaging; the fresh leaf can be used as a poultice or in a compress. Soothes inflamed wounds or sores.
- Used internally to treat diarrhea, colitis, hemorrhoids, or internal bleeding.
- May be infused in oil and made into lotions or ointments to treat hemorrhoids, burns, skin ulcers, boils, eczema, or other skin irritations.
- Used as a spring tonic, and may also be eaten fresh in salads or as a potherb.
- Popular in traditional Chinese medicine, it was used to treat "liver heat," improve circulation, and lower blood pressure, and as a diuretic for kidney complaints.
- Some studies show it could be promising in treating herpes, HIV, and breast cancer, and may provide protection from sun damage due to UVA and UVB rays.
- Some claim it may be useful in regulating thyroid issues.

FOLKLORE: Was once believed to be a holy herb that could drive away the devil. Some Indigenous peoples have used it in traditional ceremonies before a hunt to sharpen their powers of concentration.

INFUSION: Infuse 1–2 tsp. dried herb in 1 cup boiling water. Steep 1 hour. Drink 3 times a day, or use as a gargle or lotion.

HOPS

Humulus lupulus

FAMILY: *Cannabaceae* (Hemp)

OTHER NAMES: Common hops, *Fr.* Houblon

PARTS USED: Fruit (cones)

CHARACTERISTICS: Bitter, cold, dry, slightly pungent

SYSTEMS AFFECTED: Nervous system

ACTIONS: Sedative, diuretic, tonic, antiseptic, nervine

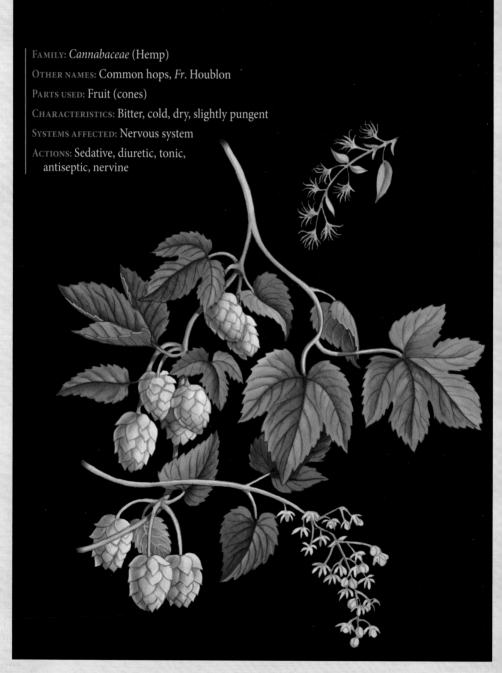

Hops may be well known as a stabilizer and bitter flavouring and natural preservative for beer, but it is also a potent medicinal herb. This climbing perennial vine, often growing up to 6 metres long, is native to North America but is also cultivated all over the world. Typically it is found growing wild along old railway sites and farmlands. The leaves are opposite, dark green, and heart-shaped with finely toothed edges; the larger ones having 3–5 sharply toothed lobes. The flowers, like hemp, grow male and female on separate plants. The male flowers grow in bunches 7.5–12 cm. long; the females grow in cone-like strobiles about 3 cm. long. Only the females are used for brewing beer and as a medicine. The strobiles are gathered when they turn an amber-brown colour, in August or September, and should be dried gently in an oven to preserve their volatile oils.

MEDICINAL USES:

Anxiety, insomnia, lack of appetite, indigestion, sluggish liver

- Dried strobiles used in infusions or put into pillows to promote sleep.
- Slightly heated, they may be used to relieve toothaches or earaches.
- Eases restlessness, headache, anxiety, nerve pain. May be added to cough syrups to calm irritable coughs.
- Has a relaxing influence over the digestive tract, relieves nervous indigestion, increases bile production, stimulates appetite, eases cramps, IBS, or mucous colitis, sluggish liver, jaundice.
- Contains estrogen-like chemicals that promote menstruation and flow of breast milk, and eases vaginal dryness or discomforts of menopause.
- When combined with Chamomile flowers and applied as a poultice or ointment, Hops are an effective anti-inflammatory, and can relieve pain from swelling, bruises, and boils. For rheumatic pains and neuralgia, apply as a hot poultice.
- Antiviral activity means it could have an effect on herpes, HIV, and certain cancers.
- Believed by some to encourage hair growth.
- Clinical trials showed a decrease in blood–glucose levels in patients with Type 2 diabetes.

INFUSION: Add 2 tsp dried hops to 1 cup of boiling water. Steep for 5 minutes. For insomnia, add Valerian and/or Passionflower.

IMPORTANT: May aggravate feelings of depression in people with low energy and anxiety. Frequent contact may cause dermatitis in some people.

HORSETAIL

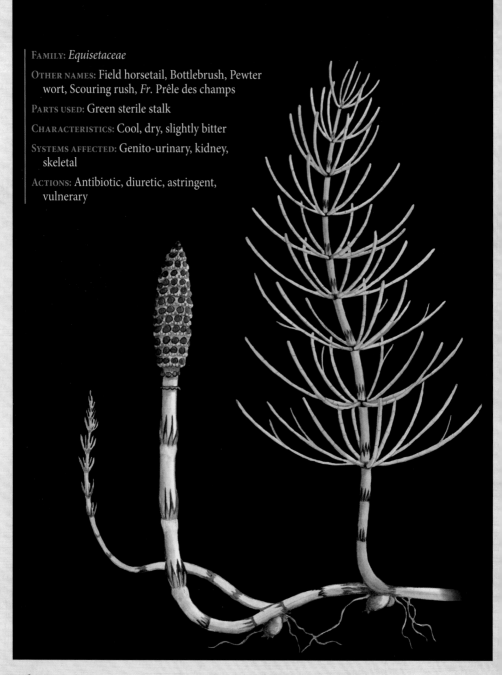

Equisetum arvense

FAMILY: *Equisetaceae*

OTHER NAMES: Field horsetail, Bottlebrush, Pewter wort, Scouring rush, *Fr.* Prêle des champs

PARTS USED: Green sterile stalk

CHARACTERISTICS: Cool, dry, slightly bitter

SYSTEMS AFFECTED: Genito-urinary, kidney, skeletal

ACTIONS: Antibiotic, diuretic, astringent, vulnerary

Horsetail is a rather odd-looking, prehistoric-like, non-flowering native plant. It reproduces by spores, which are located under the scales of the asparagus-like shoot, a spike of around 20 cm. tall, which appears in the spring. In summer the spike disappears and is replaced by a green sterile stalk with whorls of thin branches, resembling a smaller version of the large tree-like plants that covered the earth 400 million years ago. These stems and branches contain silicon crystals, which makes it useful for cleaning and polishing metal objects or kitchen utensils. It is usually found in swamps, damp woods, and fields.

MEDICINAL USES:

Urinary tract infections, osteoporosis, joint problems, wounds, kidney and bladder disorders

- Traditionally used as a diuretic to increase urine output and relieve chronic urinary tract infections and kidney stones. Helps cure incontinence and bedwetting.
- Astringent, it tightens and tones tissue in cases of diarrhea, hemorrhoids, and dysentery.
- Crushed sterile stems used as a poultice will stop bleeding and heal cuts, sores, and other wounds. Stops hemorrhaging.
- Reduces inflammation of the prostate.
- Because of the presence of silica, a mineral essential to bone health, it strengthens and heals joints and bones. Some have suggested it may be useful as a treatment for osteoporosis; however, there is no scientific evidence as yet.
- Dissolved in the bath, it can be soothing for rheumatic pain, rashes, or other wounds. In a foot bath, it can help ease infections.
- Liquid obtained from boiling stems often used as a mouthwash or gargle to treat oral infections, cankers, or sore throat. Add salt if desired.
- A few drops of tincture mixed with coconut oil helps keeps hair shiny, strengthens brittle nails, and prevents signs of aging skin.

OTHER USES: As an abrasive for scouring pots and pans or polishing metal.

BATH SOAK: Steep ½ cup horsetail in hot water for 1 hour. Add liquid to bathwater.

COMPRESS: Crush dried herb and mix in enough warm water to form a paste. Mix with crushed Plantain if desired. Apply to boils or other sores 2 times a day.

INFUSION: Mix 2 tsp. dried herb in 1 cup boiling water, steep for 15 minutes. Strain. Drink 3 times a day. Can be mixed with lemon juice and/or salt to be used as a gargle.

IMPORTANT: Avoid internal use for more than 1 week at a time. Do not exceed recommended dosage. Do not use if you are diabetic or have a deficiency in thiamine or potassium, as its diuretic properties may deplete these nutrients. Avoid if pregnant or breastfeeding.

HYSSOP

Hyssopus officinalis

FAMILY: *Lamiaceae*

OTHER NAMES: *Fr.* Hysope

PARTS USED: Aerial, dried

CHARACTERISTICS: Bitter, pungent, dry, slightly warming

SYSTEMS AFFECTED: Lungs, stomach

ACTIONS: Demulcent, antispasmodic, antiseptic, expectorant, diaphoretic, sedative, carminative, aromatic, tonic, vulnerary

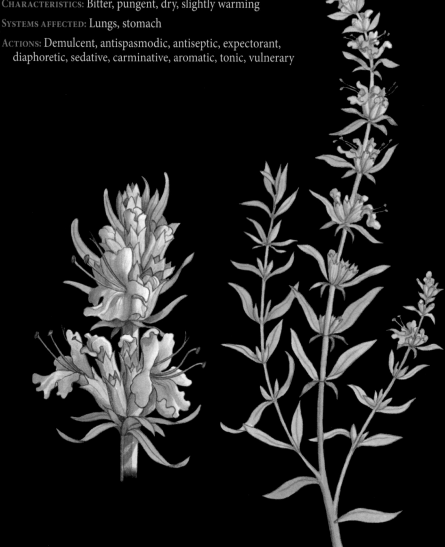

Hyssop is an aromatic shrubby perennial that grows in clumps along fields and roadsides throughout the summer. It has stalks growing up to 60 cm. tall with shiny dark-green opposite-toothed leaves along a square stem and many tiny 2-lipped purple flowers that run up one side of the top part of the erect stalk. It has been used since ancient times for ritual cleaning of sacred places because of its unusual odour, and when planted in a garden, it attracts bees and butterflies. Harvest in August when in flower.

MEDICINAL USES:

Respiratory ailments, indigestion

- Tea mainly used for respiratory problems, especially bronchitis, but also used to treat colds, inflammation of the chest and throat, or unproductive coughs with thick mucus. Relaxes and loosens when used along with drinking plenty of water. Best used as a tonic after the worst of the infection has passed.
- Tea made from the leaves may also be used to ease flatulence and/or stomachache.
- Improves circulation; poultice made from the fresh herb is used to heal wounds, and infusions of the fresh leaves can be applied to ease the pain of rheumatism.
- The essential oil of Hyssop is widely used in aromatherapy and can be diluted, added to bathwater, or added to coconut oil and used to treat skin problems, rheumatism, indigestion, fevers, cramps, and hemorrhoids.

OTHER USES:
- Fresh flowers and young shoots may be eaten in salads.
- Crushed dried leaves and flowers may be used in potpourris or as a strewing herb to mask odours.

FOLKLORE: Once believed to be a holy plant, Hyssop was said to purify and forgive one's sins. It was also used to disinfect against the plague.

COMPRESS: 2 tbsp. dried herb mixed with 2 cups of boiling water, steep for 15 minutes. Soak a clean cloth in liquid and apply to skin.

INFUSION: Mix 2 tsp. dried herb per cup of boiling water; steep 10 minutes. Drink up to 3 times a day. Add sugar or honey if desired.

IMPORTANT: Should not be used by pregnant women as it can cause a miscarriage. Essential oil should not be used by people with a history of epilepsy. Do not exceed recommended doses.

JAPANESE KNOTWEED

Fallopia japonica

FAMILY: *Polygonaceae*

OTHER NAMES: Hu zhang, American bamboo, Fleeceflower, *Fr.* Renouée de japon

PARTS USED: Roots, rhizome, young stalks

CHARACTERISTICS: Bitter, cold, dry

ACTIONS: Analgesic, antiarthritic, antioxidant, antibacterial, anticancer, antiviral, laxative, tonic

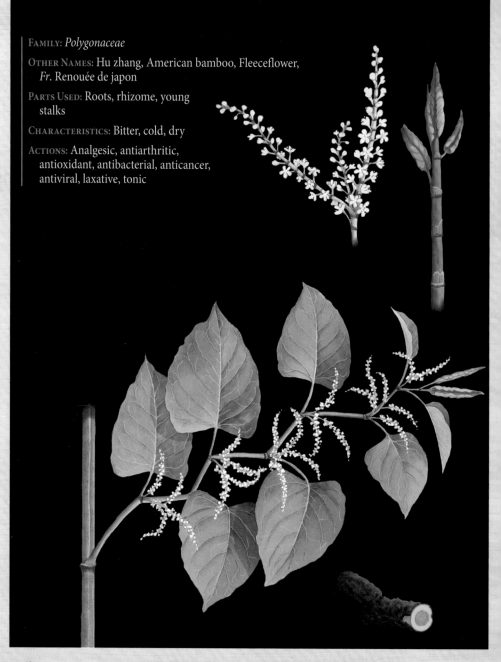

Japanese knotweed is a tenacious weed that has become a real problem in Atlantic Canada because of its invasive tendencies and resilience. A native of Japan and East Asia, it was brought to North America in the late 1800s, and quickly spread across the continent. Growing to a height of up to 3 metres with a root system that can break through concrete and extend up to 3 metres deep underground, it crowds out native plants, alters the ecosystem, and can be very difficult to remove.

It does have some redeeming qualities, however. For one thing, it tastes good. The young stems, resembling crimson asparagus, appear in April or May and are tart and crunchy, somewhat like rhubarb. It is also a valuable medicinal herb. Its root is high in resveratrol, which is important in brain function and heart health. There has also been some promising research into its use as a treatment for Lyme disease. It grows along roadsides and streams, and has a bright green hollow stalk with red dividing the sections of growth, somewhat like bamboo. The heart-shaped leaves are flat at the base and emerge from these points, its veins red when young and lighter as it matures. Harvest the young stems before they turn woody; the roots may be dug up in the spring as the shoots are beginning to appear, and should be sliced thinly and tinctured or dried before use.

MEDICINAL USES:

Dementia, heart disease, Lyme disease, gingivitis

- Contains high amounts of resveratrol, which may help slow the aging process and prevent neurodegeneration. This could keep brain pathways functioning properly and perhaps ultimately prevent dementia and Alzheimer's—but clinical research has yet to demonstrate medical efficacy. It lowers cholesterol, modulates blood pressure, is anti-inflammatory, and could lower the risk of heart attack and stroke, promoting healthy circulation.
- Relieves constipation, bloating, and many other digestive issues; soothes inflammation.
- Regulates insulin and blood sugar levels.
- Effective against Lyme disease, it is part of a protocol that supports the immune system and kills the spirochetes hiding in areas of the body antibiotics can't reach.
- As a mouthwash, helpful against gingivitis; decreases bleeding and formation of plaque.
- Some studies show promise in preventing and treating certain types of cancer.
- Helps to detoxify the liver and heal wounds, and helps relieve symptoms of gout and rheumatoid arthritis.

DECOCTION: Mix 1 tsp. of dried root in 1 cup of water; simmer 10 minutes. Let stand to steep for half an hour. Take ½ cup 2 times a day.

IMPORTANT: Avoid taking in large amounts as it could cause nausea and vomiting. Do not use with blood-thinning medications. Do not use during pregnancy.

JEWELWEED

Impatiens capensis

FAMILY: *Balsaminaceae*

OTHER NAMES: Wild Balsam, Orange jewelweed, Spotted touch-me-not, Slipperweed, *Fr.* Impatiente du Cap, Chou Sauvage

PARTS USED: Aerial

SYSTEMS AFFECTED: Skin

ACTIONS: Antidote, anti-inflammatory, cathartic, diuretic, emetic, fungicide

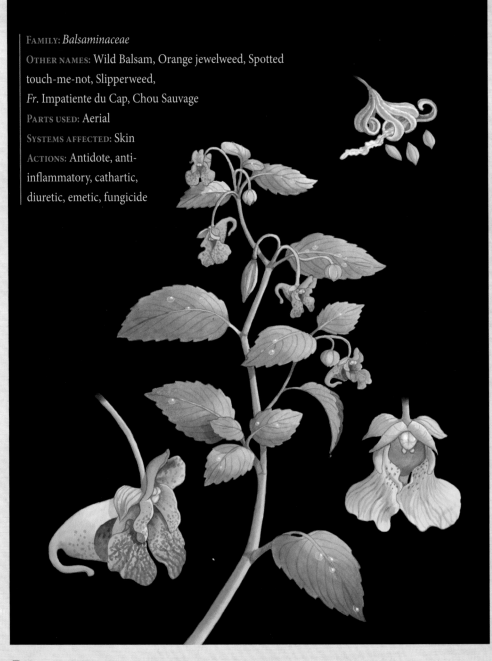

This delicate annual grows throughout the summer in low-lying, damp soil, often close to streams. Easily recognizable by its small, orange, trumpet-shaped flowers with curved tails and darker spots inside, it is one of the best remedies for Poison Ivy, and often grows nearby. The stems are long and tender, growing in clumps that can be 1 metre or more tall, and the leaves are thin, ovate, and slightly toothed. The leaves will repel water, giving it its name, as water will bead up into tiny jewel-like droplets. The ripe oblong seed pods will explode when touched, scattering its seeds and giving it the name "touch-me-not." There is another species of Jewelweed, *Impatiens pallida*, which has yellow flowers and has similar medicinal properties, but is less potent than the orange variety. It is an attractive plant for hummingbirds and butterflies.

MEDICINAL USES:

Skin irritations

- Fresh juice of the stem and leaves contains balsaminones, which relieve itch and irritation from Poison Ivy, Poison Oak, or Nettles.
- Potent anti-fungal and anti-inflammatory properties make it effective in treating athlete's foot and fungal dermatitis. A poultice of the leaves can be applied to bruises, cuts, burns, eczema, acne, or insect bites. Also effective treatment for warts and corns.
- In a salve or ointment, it can be used to relieve the itch of hemorrhoids.

OTHER USES: Yellow dye can be made from the flowers.

TREATMENT FOR SKIN IRRITATIONS: Fill a stockpot with chopped fresh jewelweed, cover with water, and boil until water is reduced by half. Strain and pour into ice cube trays. Freeze and use as needed. Good for up to 1 year.

IMPORTANT: Herb has an acrid burning taste and can act as an emetic and purgative. Internal use not recommended. Does not dry well. Not recommended for use in tinctures, as some people have a bad reaction when jewelweed is mixed with alcohol.

LABRADOR TEA

Rhododendron groenlandicum (Ledum groenlandicum)

FAMILY: *Ericaceae*

OTHER NAMES: Bog Labrador Tea, Muskeg Tea, *Fr.* Thé du Labrador, Lédon de Groenland

PARTS USED: Leaves, flowers

CHARACTERISTICS: Spicy, fragrant

SYSTEMS AFFECTED: Kidneys, liver

ACTIONS: Tonic, diaphoretic, astringent, analgesic, diuretic, narcotic, insecticide, anti-inflammatory

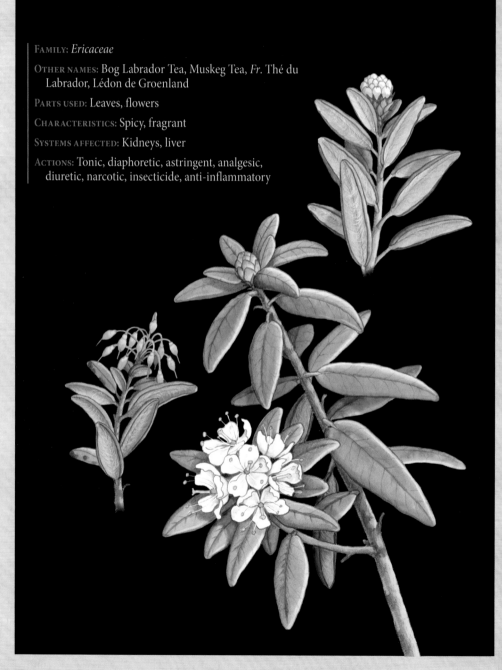

Labrador Tea is a native evergreen shrub that has long been used by Indigenous peoples as a soothing tea and medicine, and by European settlers as a tea replacement during shortages. It grows in bogs, moist forests, and along roadsides to a height of up to 1.5 metres with alternate elliptical leaves that are green and leathery on top, and rusty coloured and woolly underneath. The leaves droop slightly on the branch, and their edges are rolled under. In June and July tiny clusters of white flowers form on the end of each hairy stalk. The leaves are best if collected in the spring just before the flowers open.

MEDICINAL PROPERTIES:

Respiratory infections, skin irritations, diabetes, headaches, kidney ailments

- Fragrant and soothing tea used for centuries by many northern Indigenous peoples. Helps with respiratory infections, coughs, sore throat, bronchitis. Some women use it shortly before giving birth, as it is mildly narcotic. Use with caution: do not boil, and only brew for a short time in an open container, or change the water halfway through the steeping process.
- The Mi'kmaq use the tea to treat kidney ailments and stones, and as a tonic and blood purifier. The Cree use it as an anti-diabetic medicine, and it has been shown to lower blood glucose levels and improve insulin levels.
- Soothes headaches, asthma, colds, and indigestion.
- A stronger decoction made from the powdered leaves or root can be used externally as a wash for burns, skin irritations, and chapped skin, or made into an ointment.

OTHER USES:
- Leaves strewn in closets keep moths away.
- Tincture used to kill lice, mosquitoes, and fleas; repels mice.
- Brown dye can be obtained from plant.
- Used as flavouring in stews and marinades.

INFUSION: Put 2 tsp. herb (fresh or dried) into a pot and cover with 4 cups of water. Bring to a boil until the water turns light green. Strain out coloured water and add another 4 cups of fresh water to the pot, bringing it back to a boil. When the water turns yellow, strain into a teapot and drink no more than 2 cups per day.

IMPORTANT: Do not boil tea if using internally. Brew for only a short period of time in an open container. Not recommended if pregnant or breastfeeding. Do not consume in excess, as it is slightly narcotic and can cause headaches and/or vomiting in large doses.

LADY'S MANTLE

Alchemilla glabra (Smooth)
A. vulgaris (Thinstem)
A. monticola (Hairy)

FAMILY: *Rosaceae*

OTHER NAMES: Dew-cup, Lion's Foot, Bear's Foot, *Fr.* Alchémille,
Pied-de-Lion

PARTS USED: Leaves and flowers

CHARACTERISTICS: Bitter, astringent, slightly
warm, dry

SYSTEMS AFFECTED: Kidneys, uterus

ACTIONS: Astringent,
depurative,
emmenagogue, tonic,
vulnerary

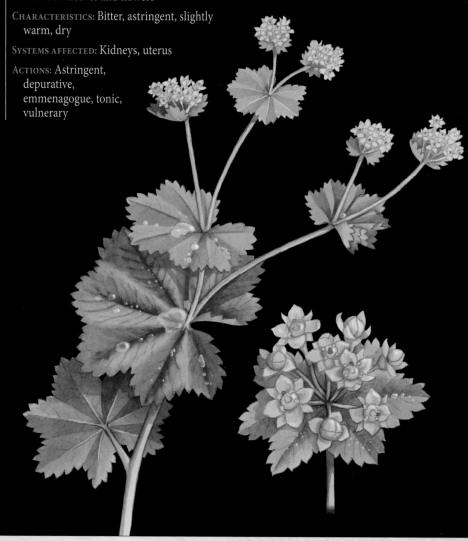

This small, inconspicuous plant is found in cool and wet climates around the world, but in eastern Canada most are found in cultivated gardens or have escaped into the wild. It gets its name from the Arab word "alkemelych," meaning alchemy, which refers to the belief that the dewdrops that beaded up on its leaves hold magical powers of transformation. It is a perennial with an erect stem standing about 30 cm. high. The lower kidney-shaped leaves have 7 or 9 lobes, and are finely toothed at the edges; upper leaves are notched and toothed and folded somewhat like a fan. The small green/yellow flowers grow in clusters from June to August. The whole plant is covered with soft tiny hairs. The leaves and flowers should be gathered early in the summer and dried for later use.

MEDICINAL USES:

Heavy menstruation, wounds, prolapsed uterus, childbirth, arthritis, vaginitis

- Strong astringent, it contains bitters, salicylic acid, tannins, and vitamin C, and is used to dry up tissues, relieve diarrhea, colitis, and leukorrhea, stop hemorrhage and infection in wounds with inflammation. Dries, cleans, tones, and strengthens skin and tissues. Use a compress soaked in tea made from the herb.
- Has a beneficial effect on the female reproductive system, toning tissues and muscles just before or after childbirth or other trauma to the uterus (abortion, miscarriage, surgery, etc.). Strengthens the womb, treats symptoms of vaginitis, candida, and heavy menstrual bleeding. Combined with Yarrow, it establishes regular menstrual cycles in young girls suffering from heavy bleeding and irregular periods. When taken with Raspberry leaf for about 3 weeks, it can be useful in treating a prolapsed uterus.
- Restores strength to torn, ruptured tissues (hernias, perforated eardrums).
- For arthritis and gout, dries dampness in the joints, relieves pain—use in an oil and apply externally.
- Strengthens and tones muscles when atrophy has occurred, as in MS, weak heart, or prolapse.

FOLKLORE: This plant's name was once associated with the Virgin Mary, and dewdrops that gathered on its leaves were used in potions. The herb placed under a pillow at night was said to promote a good night's sleep.

INFUSION: Mix 2 tsp. dried herb in 1 cup of boiling water; infuse 10–15 minutes. Drink 3 times a day. Add Raspberry leaf or Shepherd's Purse for excess bleeding or to tone tissues.

TINCTURE: Start with 1–2 ml. 3 times a day, and increase if necessary.

IMPORTANT: Do not use during the early stages of pregnancy, as it is a uterine stimulant and could cause miscarriage. Do not exceed recommended dose. Avoid use 2 weeks before or after surgery.

LEMON BALM

Melissa officinalis

FAMILY: *Lamiaceae*

OTHER NAMES: Melissa, Balm, Sweet Balm, *Fr.* Mélisse

PARTS USED: Leaves

CHARACTERISTICS: Sour, spicy, cool

SYSTEMS AFFECTED: Lungs, liver

ACTIONS: Diaphoretic, calmative, anti-viral, antispasmodic, carminative, emmenagogue, stomachic, febrifuge, nervine

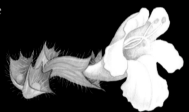

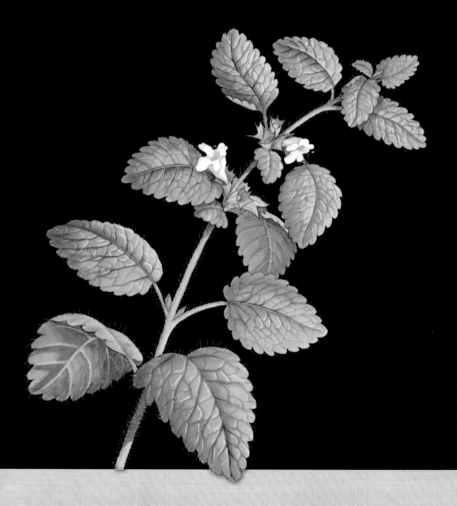

A native of Europe, this perennial now grows all over the world, although here in eastern Canada it is mostly found in cultivated gardens rather than in the wild. The scientific name *Melissa* stems from the Greek word for honey, and the plant was likely so named because of bees' attraction to it. It grows from 30 to 60 cm. high and has fine hairs. The leaves are opposite, oval, and wrinkled, with scalloped edges, and give off a pleasant lemony scent when rubbed. The stem is square and branched, and the flowers appear in small bunches around the leaf axils from June to October. The plant dies down in winter, but the root is perennial. Harvest in the afternoon in early summer when the oils are strongest. Best if tinctured fresh.

MEDICINAL USES:

Stress, insomnia, indigestion, wounds, cold sores

- Has a tonic effect on the heart, slightly lowering blood pressure and easing tension, depression, anxiety, palpitations. Research in clinical studies shows that Lemon Balm is effective in helping promote sleep, particularly when added to other sleep-inducing herbs. Relieves muscle spasms, increases calmness and alertness, and improves memory.
- Soothes upset stomach, especially where there is anxiety. Relieves gas and promotes appetite.
- Indigenous peoples have traditionally used Lemon Balm in preparations to treat colds, fever, and chills, as it induces perspiration.
- Used in ointments to prevent and relieve cold sores, herpes lesions, and ulcers, to heal open wounds, and to stop bleeding.
- Leaves steeped in wine were once used to relieve reactions to insect bites and stings.

INFUSION: Mix 1 tsp. dried herb in 1 cup of boiling water. Drink up to 4 times a day, or after meals. For insomnia, add Valerian. For cold sores steep 2–4 tsp. crushed herb in 1 cup boiling water. Cool and apply with cotton swabs throughout the day.

TINCTURE: 60 drops daily.

CALMING TEA:
- 4 parts Lemon Balm
- 3 parts Chamomile
- 2 parts Skullcap
- 1 part Motherwort
- Use 2–3 tsp. per 1 cup boiling water. Steep for 10 minutes.

IMPORTANT: May interact with sedatives, certain thyroid medications, or drugs for HIV. Consult your doctor if you are taking any medications.

MARSHMALLOW

Altheae officinalis

FAMILY: *Malvaceae*

OTHER NAMES: White mallow, *Fr.* Guimauve

PARTS USED: Leaf, flowers, root

CHARACTERISTICS: Cool, moist, sweet

SYSTEMS AFFECTED: Lungs, stomach

ACTIONS: Demulcent, alterative, diuretic, vulnerary, mild laxative, emollient, expectorant, antibacterial, anti-inflammatory

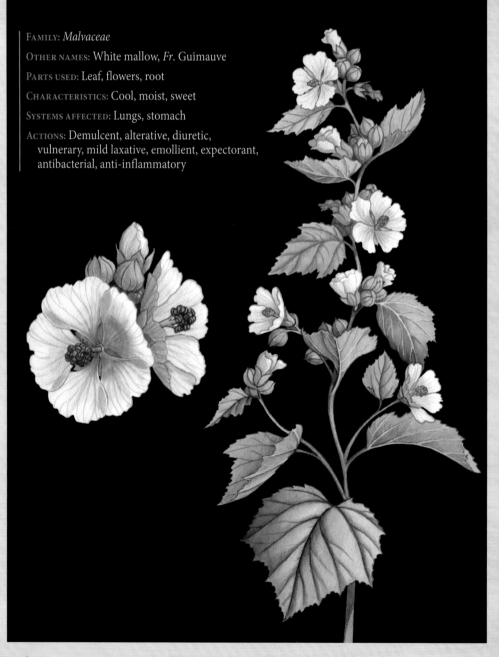

This tall perennial has been used for centuries all over the world as a vegetable, but is also one of the most treasured healing herbs available. The treats we buy today with the same name no longer contain any trace of the plant, but in the early 1800s in France, there was a confection called Paté de Guimauve, which was a spongy square made from the plant's gooey root sap along with whipped egg whites and sugar that eventually evolved into our modern campfire treat.

The erect stems can be up to 1.5 metres tall, with alternate, irregular-toothed leaves that are soft and velvety on both sides. The round flowers are pale pink or white with a darker pink centre and 5 petals each. The roots are white and mucilaginous, tasting somewhat like parsnip. It typically thrives in damp places, such as marshes—as its name suggests—but is now almost exclusively grown in the dry soil of cultivated gardens. Plants should be at least 2 years old before using as medicine. Flowers are best used just as they are coming into bloom in mid- to late summer. Leaves should be picked on a dry day and the root should be harvested in the fall.

MEDICINAL USES:

Soothes mucous membranes of digestive, urinary, and respiratory tracts; reduces skin inflammation

- Because of its mucilaginous properties, an infusion made from the leaves can help relieve a dry cough, asthma, and bronchitis, as well as soothing the mucous membranes of the throat and mouth, forming a protective layer over inflamed tissue. The flowers can also be used to make a cough syrup.
- A cold decoction of the root eases heartburn, indigestion, ulcers, and since the mucilage reaches the colon, it can help with ulcerative colitis and Crohn's disease. Mix with peppermint or Ginger for a soothing tea.
- The root is also good if taken as a decoction at the first sign of cystitis to speed healing.
- A peeled root may be used as a chew stick for teething infants.
- Powdered dry or crushed fresh roots can be used externally in a warm poultice for skin irritations, boils, burns, sores, and minor wounds; reduces inflammation and speeds healing. Added to creams or salves to treat eczema or contact dermatitis. Fresh leaves may be applied to bee stings.

COLD DECOCTION: Soak 2 tbsp. Marshmallow root (fresh or dried) in cold water for half an hour, then peel and cut into small pieces. Let peeled root stand in the water for another 2 hours. Sweeten mixture with honey and drink lukewarm. Good for coughs, indigestion.

IMPORTANT: Marshmallow tends to coat the stomach lining so it may interfere with absorption of other herbs or drugs. Best taken several hours before or after taking other medications. May decrease blood sugar. Talk to a doctor before taking if you have diabetes.

MILK THISTLE

Silybum marianum

FAMILY: *Asteraceae*

OTHER NAMES: St. Mary's Thistle, *Fr.* Chardon-marie

PARTS USED: Seeds, leaves, root

CHARACTERISTICS: Bland, slightly bitter

SYSTEMS AFFECTED: Liver, spleen, kidneys

ACTIONS: Antioxidant, anti-inflammatory, astringent, cholagogue, diaphoretic, diuretic, galactagogue

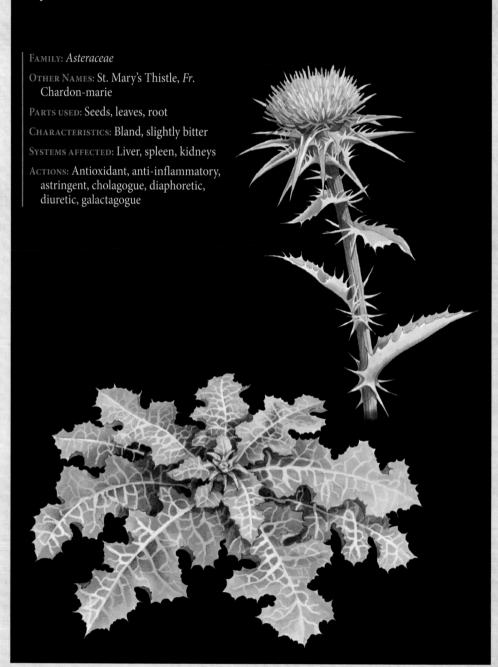

Milk Thistle, or St. Mary's Thistle, has been used for thousands of years throughout Europe and the Middle East as a liver remedy. Large and distinctive, its spiny leaves are marbled with white veins that were said to be the milk of the Virgin Mary, hence its name. It can grow up to 1.5 metres tall, and its magenta-coloured flowers appear at the top of the stems from April to October. Spiny bracts surround the flowers and give them a star-like appearance. It's considered a noxious weed in some areas, as it can be toxic to cattle and sheep, especially when grown in nitrate-rich soil. It should be harvested only from organic areas that have not been used for farmland or treated with pesticides.

MEDICINAL USES:

Liver, spleen and kidney congestion, mushroom poisoning, alcohol and drug abuse, low milk production

- One of the best liver remedies available, it contains silymarin, which has been studied extensively and proven to be effective in regenerating liver cells and protecting them from poisons. Used to reduce the toxic effects of alcohol or drug abuse, junk food, chemical pollution, or other threats to normal liver function. Can reduce the toxicity of Amanita mushroom poisoning.
- Its antioxidants increase the resiliency of liver cells and encourage new growth. It stimulates bile, relieves congestion in the liver, spleen, and kidneys, reduces inflammation in the gallbladder, and assists in digestion of fats.
- Symptoms of poor liver function may include poor skin or itching, food allergies, digestive problems, cold, dry constitution, constipation with small, hard, dry stool, and gallstones.
- Increases milk flow for lactating women; safe for use during pregnancy.

OTHER USES: All parts are edible, however the thorns need to be removed from each leaf. 1–2 tsp. ground seeds per day may be added to smoothies. Reduce dose if it causes diarrhea.

TINCTURE: Take 5–60 drops, depending on severity of the condition.

IMPORTANT: Generally safe, but use only organic herb from a reputable dealer as it has a tendency to absorb nitrates from fertilized farmland.

MILKWEED

Asclepias syriaca (Common)
Asclepias incarnate (Swamp)

FAMILY: *Apocynaceae*

OTHER NAMES: Common silkweed, Swamp Milkweed, Cottonweed, Wild Cotton, *Fr.* Laiteron, Cochons de lait

PARTS USED: Whole plant

SYSTEMS AFFECTED: Lungs

ACTIONS: Diuretic, anodyne, emetic, purgative, alterative, tonic, diaphoretic, expectorant (roots also emmenagogue)

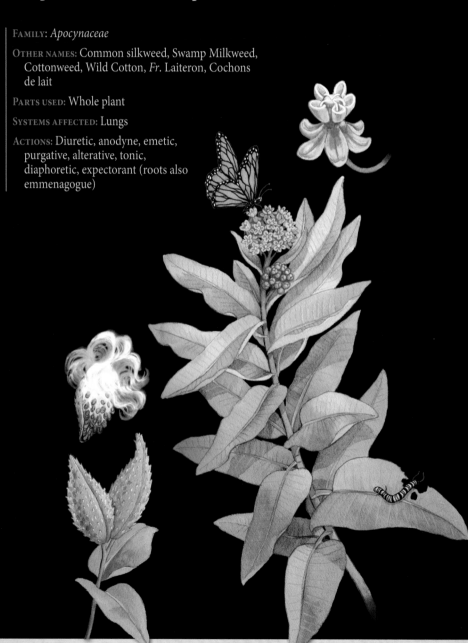

The name Milkweed comes from the thick milky sap or latex that oozes from the plant when cut. It is a native perennial with a thick, hollow unbranched stem that grows 1–2 metres tall. The large, leathery, opposite leaves are smooth on top and downy underneath. The umbels of the terminal or lateral flowers are fragrant and pink or purplish, blooming from July to August. They are followed by the growth of fleshy seed pods, which are about 5–12 cm. long, grey-green and warty with prickles, and contain a wad of feathery down and flat brown seeds arranged in overlapping rows. Milkweed can be found in fields and along roadsides and is a favourite of the Monarch butterfly larvae, which chew the leaves to make themselves distasteful to predators. Grazing animals usually avoid Milkweed, as it can be toxic for them. Harvest roots in the fall and dry. Be careful not to confuse with Butterfly Weed, which has bright orange flowers, clear sap, and is inedible. Dogbane, which is poisonous, is also similar but the stem is solid, reddish, often branched, and has a bitter taste.

MEDICINAL USES:

Coughs, skin ailments

- Indigenous peoples use the sap to treat skin problems such as Poison Ivy rash and ringworm. To remove warts, the fresh sap should be applied several times a day over a few weeks until the wart disappears. The plant can also be used externally on eczema, burns, sores, and wounds.
- Infusions of the roots and leaves can be used for suppressing coughs, and treating asthma, bronchitis, and pleurisy. It relaxes the bronchioles, reduces coughing and spasms, and liquefies mucus in the lungs. Some Indigenous peoples use it in a powdered root tea to treat sexually transmitted infections, as a laxative or sedative, to cause vomiting and/or expel worms.
- Strong diaphoretic, induces sweating to bring down a fever, also stimulates circulation to the extremities in cases of poor circulation and edema (swelling).
- Stems can be cooked and applied to joints to treat rheumatism.

OTHER USES:
- Young Milkweed sprouts resemble asparagus and are edible, as are the young seed pods, but all parts should be cooked for 10 minutes in water and drained before eating to remove the toxic compounds. Unopened flower buds can be boiled and eaten like peas, and the flower clusters boiled down to obtain a brown sugar.
- The plant was once cultivated for its silky down from the seed pods to use in life jackets and to stuff beds and pillows. Recently, cultivation has been revived in Quebec to provide insulation for winter coats.
- The stem's tough stringy fibres can be made into rope or woven into a coarse fabric.

IMPORTANT: Milkweed contains small amounts of toxic cardio-active glycosides. Not for use if you have a heart condition or high blood pressure. Not for use during pregnancy. Older leaves are poisonous if consumed in large quantities or over a long period of time. Use recommended only by a certified herbalist or in formulas not exceeding 25%. Do not get sap in eyes; wash hands thoroughly after handling.

MINT

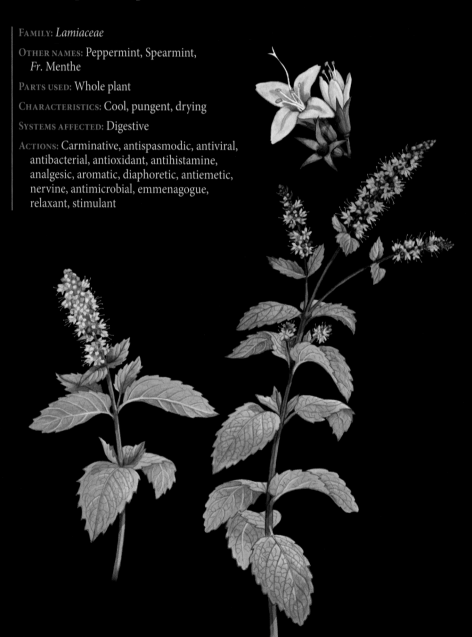

Mentha x piperita (Peppermint)
Mentha spicata (Spearmint)

FAMILY: *Lamiaceae*

OTHER NAMES: Peppermint, Spearmint,
Fr. Menthe

PARTS USED: Whole plant

CHARACTERISTICS: Cool, pungent, drying

SYSTEMS AFFECTED: Digestive

ACTIONS: Carminative, antispasmodic, antiviral,
antibacterial, antioxidant, antihistamine,
analgesic, aromatic, diaphoretic, antiemetic,
nervine, antimicrobial, emmenagogue,
relaxant, stimulant

Mint is a well-known invasive perennial that is easily identified by its familiar cooling aroma and taste. There are hundreds of varieties, but the two most popular are probably Peppermint (*M. x piperita*), a hybrid between Spearmint and Watermint and the one usually used in herbal medicine; and Spearmint (*M. spicata*), although many others grow wild in eastern Canada. They are visually similar but with a slightly different taste and odour. Both grow up to just under 1 metre tall, with square stems and runners that spread quickly if not confined. They prefer damp, moist soils and have toothed oblong leaves. The flowers are pink, mauve, or white, and grow in spikes throughout the summer. Harvest when the plants are in bloom and have the most flavour.

MEDICINAL USES:

Indigestion, upper respiratory ailments, colds and flu, sore muscles

- Has an analgesic and anesthetic effect on the nervous system and is an antioxidant, antiviral, and antimicrobial. May possibly have anti-tumor properties. Has a significant antihistamine effect on allergies.
- Infusion relieves bloating and stomach and intestinal gas caused by overeating; stimulates the bile and digestive juices. Has a relaxing effect on gastrointestinal tissue, relieving cramping and muscle spasms in the gastrointestinal tract. One or two drops of essential oil on a sugar cube or in water can relieve colic or IBS in children and ease the symptoms of Crohn's and ulcerative colitis. Combines well with Ginger or Liquorice root for digestive disorders.
- Essential oils may be used in balms for upper respiratory ailments, and as a soothing rub to relieve sore muscles and rheumatism. It is also a decongestant and can be used to treat headache and tension when rubbed on the temples.
- An infusion of equal parts Peppermint herb and Elder flowers (with the addition of either Boneset or Yarrow if desired) will get rid of a cold within 36 hours, according to Maud Grieve's 1931 book, *A Modern Herbal*.

OTHER USES:
- Leaves were once scattered around the house to repel vermin and rid the place of foul odours.
- Flavouring in toothpaste, candies, and beverages.

IMPORTANT: People with gallbladder issues, acid reflux, or problems with the esophagus should avoid this herb. Peppermint essential oil is highly concentrated and should be used with caution as it may cause dermatitis—dilute before consuming. Overconsumption may cause relaxing of the peristaltic action of the colon, slowing the movement of food in the GI tract. Do not take if you have a hiatal hernia. Avoid if breastfeeding, as it may dry up milk supply.

MOTHERWORT

Leonurus cardiaca

FAMILY: *Lamiaceae*

OTHER NAMES: Lion's Tail, Heartwort, *Fr.* Agripaume

PARTS USED: Leaves and flowers

CHARACTERISTICS: Bitter, spicy, cool, pungent

SYSTEMS AFFECTED: Cardiovascular, liver, uterus, nervous system

ACTIONS: Analgesic, sedative, emmenagogue, antispasmodic, cardiac tonic, hypotensive, nervine, diuretic, carminative, astringent, anti-inflammatory, aperient, febrifuge, diaphoretic, antidepressant

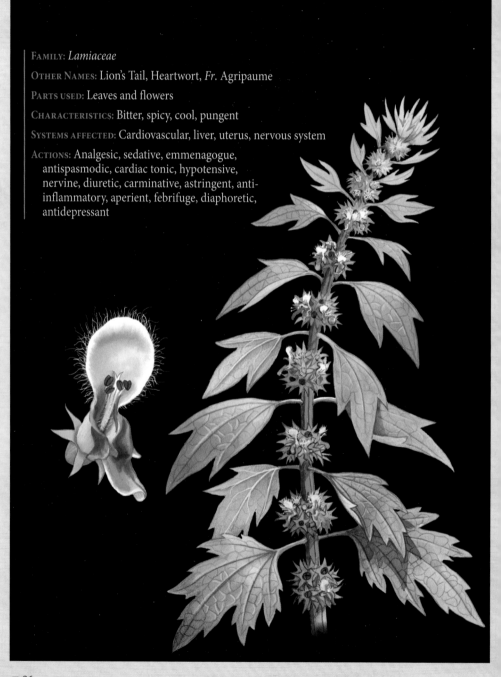

Motherwort is a perennial plant native to continental Europe. It has been grown since medieval times for its effectiveness in dealing with anxiety and "female disorders" (which then would have included childbirth, menopause, menstruation, and "hysteria"), and even to promote longevity. It grows wild throughout Eastern Canada (except for Newfoundland), and thrives in humus-rich soil and bright sun. It can be cultivated from seeds or by root propagation in spring or fall. The erect, square stems are up to 1.5 metres tall, and are often red and slightly hairy. The leaves are opposite and have 3–5 pointed lobes, also slightly hairy, and greyish on the underside. The 3-lobed flowers appear in July or August and are pink or purplish, hairy, and grow in clusters at the leaf axils. Motherwort may be collected when it blooms, before the seeds are formed, and dried for later use. Make sure to leave part of the stalk so as not to kill the plant.

MEDICINAL USES:

Suppressed or painful menstruation, arteriosclerosis, angina, palpitations, stress-related conditions

- Fresh herb tincture preferred; fresh or dried herb used in infusions, poultices, ointments, or infused oil. Particularly suited for people with anxiety, depression, palpitations, and mood swings.
- Brings on suppressed menstruation, especially due to anxiety or tension; relieves blood congestion, cramps, and painful periods. Excellent tonic for female reproductive system.
- Heart tonic, it reduces hypertension, improves blood circulation, dissolves blood clots, relieves angina on effort and palpitations. Strengthens and improves the heart when combined with Valerian root and Hawthorn.
- Helps insomnia, calms the nerves, and may work as an antidepressant and/or sedative. Combines well with Ginko, St. John's Wort, Lavender, Passionflower, Lemon Balm, Skullcap.
- Relieves pain during childbirth, promotes uterine contractions, relieves false labour pains, and helps tone the uterus and bring it back to normal after birth. May be combined with Raspberry leaf.
- Eases migraines, aids menopausal changes, and lessens anxiety.

INFUSION: 1 tsp. dried or 2 tsp. fresh herb infused in 1 cup boiling water for 5 minutes; drink 2–4 times a day.

TINCTURE: Take 10–20 drops 3 times a day.

IMPORTANT: Do not use during pregnancy, except during or after childbirth, as it can expedite the birthing process, and use only under the supervision of a midwife or doula. Do not use if you have heavy menstrual bleeding, have blood-clotting disorders, or are taking anti-coagulants. May cause dermatitis in some individuals.

MUGWORT

Artemisia vulgaris

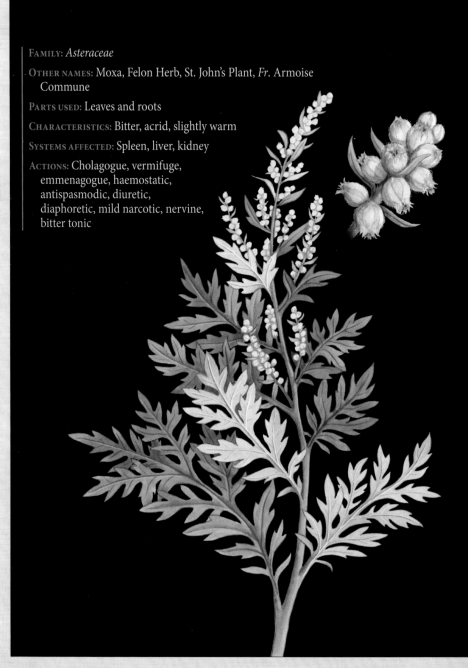

FAMILY: *Asteraceae*

OTHER NAMES: Moxa, Felon Herb, St. John's Plant, *Fr.* Armoise Commune

PARTS USED: Leaves and roots

CHARACTERISTICS: Bitter, acrid, slightly warm

SYSTEMS AFFECTED: Spleen, liver, kidney

ACTIONS: Cholagogue, vermifuge, emmenagogue, haemostatic, antispasmodic, diuretic, diaphoretic, mild narcotic, nervine, bitter tonic

Mugwort is native to Europe, Africa, and Asia, but has now spread to most parts of the world. It grows up to 1.5 metres tall and has purple stems with smooth leaves that are pointed, deeply cut, and dark green on top and woolly and silvery-coloured underneath. The flowers are cottony and yellowish-green or reddish-brown in small oval heads growing on long terminal spikes.

It can easily be mistaken for Wormwood (*Artemisia absinthium*), which looks similar and has many similar medicinal properties, but there are a few differences. Wormwood has a very bitter taste, is more silvery in colour, and is aromatic and quite bushy. Its flowers are larger and yellow when in bloom. By contrast, Mugwort has very little scent, is only slightly bitter, and is taller and more slender. The leaves and flowers should be collected just before blooming, usually in August. Cut the top third of the plant and hang to dry. The roots can be harvested in the fall and dried whole.

MEDICINAL USES:

Delayed menstruation, parasites, digestive disorders, liver problems

- Used in traditional medicine for centuries to promote menstruation and relieve cramps.
- Excellent nervine for anxiety, depression, shaking, and insomnia. Since the Middle Ages it has been used to enhance dreaming and promote sleep, although some people experience nightmares.
- Used to treat a lot of digestive complaints, including non-ulcer dyspepsia, vomiting, heartburn, cramps, and lack of appetite. Stimulates digestive juices and bile secretions, which helps digest fat and protein and relieves liver stagnation. Normalizes digestive complaints like diarrhea and constipation.
- Treats parasitic infections.
- Indigenous peoples use it to treat colds and flu, bronchitis, and fever; induces sweating.
- Used in moxibustion (burning a stick of dried, ground Mugwort onto acupuncture points of the body) to enhance treatments.
- Oil of Mugwort used topically can relieve deep muscle pain, particularly when combined with other oils like St. John's Wort. It has a soothing, warming effect on the body.

FOLKLORE: A lot of lore surrounds this herb. In ancient China and Japan, it was hung in doorways to keep disease out, and similarly used throughout Europe to ward off evil spirits. Travellers carried it on their persons to keep away wild animals and stuffed it in their shoes to alleviate fatigue. Mugwort tea was often consumed before divinations, as it was thought to be a visionary herb. Some Indigenous peoples use a Mugwort smudge to purify the air. Leaves placed under a pillow may produce lucid and colourful dreams.

INFUSION: Mix 1 tsp. dried or fresh herb in 1 cup boiling water; steep for 10 minutes. Add honey if desired.

IMPORTANT: May cause miscarriage; do not use if pregnant or breastfeeding. Not recommended for use by women who have heavy periods. May cause allergic reactions. Do not exceed recommended dosages or use for an extended period of time as it may cause pain and spasms.

MULLEIN

Verbascum thapsus

FAMILY: *Scrophulariaceae*

OTHER NAMES: White Mullein, Torches, Flannel plant, Candlewort, Candlewick, *Fr.* Bonhomme, Tabac du diable, Bouillon blanc, Molène vulgare

PARTS USED: Leaves, roots and flowers

CHARACTERISTICS: Cool, bitter, sweet, drying

SYSTEMS AFFECTED: Liver, nervous system

ACTIONS: Antiseptic, astringent, demulcent, emollient, expectorant, vulnerary

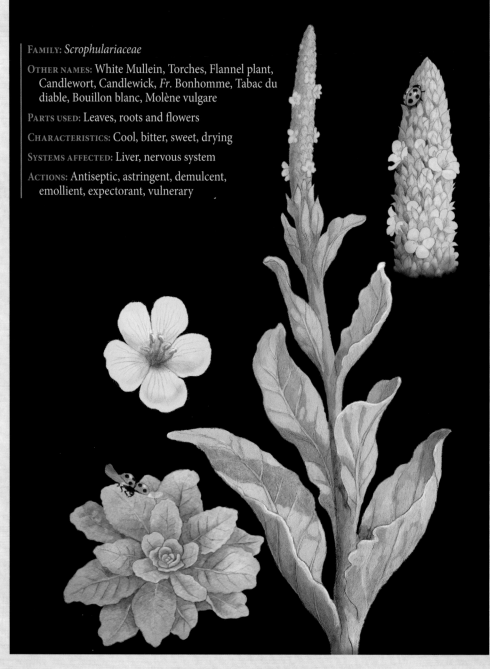

Mullein is a hard plant to miss, as it often grows to a height of 1.5 or 1.8 metres. During the first season of growth, only a rosette of soft, hairy leaves up to 38 cm. long appears. The following spring, a hairy stalk emerges from the centre, with leaves joined to the stalk and becoming smaller towards the top. The top becomes a flower spike, usually about 30 cm. long, with yellow flowers blooming randomly all along the stalk. The flowers are composed of 5 petals, each about 2.5 cm. in diameter. They should be harvested and dried quickly and carefully, so as not to bruise the delicate petals, since this will diminish their efficacy. The leaves are best when picked during the first year of growth; take only a few leaves so as not to kill the plant, and dry in the shade.

MEDICINAL USES:

Chest colds, bronchitis, asthma, earaches, and eczema

- High in mucilage, the leaves are ideal for reducing inflammation in the respiratory tract. They tone the mucous membranes, stimulate fluid production, and relax the gut wall to make expectoration easier. This works well in cases of bronchitis where there is a dry cough causing soreness. Also works to relieve symptoms of chest colds, asthma, and laryngitis. Mild sedative, it promotes sleep and calms the nerves.
- Fresh leaves work externally as a poultice to ease pain, bruising, itching, and to heal slow-healing wounds, burns, and rashes.
- Oil made by macerating flowers in olive oil is quite effective in relieving earache or eczema in the ear, as well as in treating gum and mouth ulcers. It also works on the scalp to keep it free from dandruff, helps condition hair, and when rubbed into the skin, soothes arthritis and muscle pain.
- Some Mi'kmaq have traditionally smoked the leaves to treat asthma, or steeped them in water and inhaled the vapours.

OTHER USES: Used in cosmetics to soften the skin. The leaves were once stuffed in the shoes to keep the feet warm. A yellow dye can be made from the flowers.

FOLKLORE: The stem stripped of leaves and dipped in tallow was used as a torch and to protect against enchantment. Smoked leaves were believed to clear the air of negative energies and often used in witches' ceremonies. Some people even carried the leaves to prevent conception.

INFUSION FOR COUGH: Mix 1–2 tsp. dried leaves in 1 cup of water and boil for 10 minutes. Strain thoroughly to remove any tiny hairs and plant material. Drink warm with honey. May be combined with Coltsfoot, Marshmallow, and/or Wild Thyme.

TINCTURE: Take 1–2 ml. every few hours, as needed.

EAR OIL: Dry flowers gently in a slightly warm oven until crispy, place in glass jar, cover with organic extra-virgin olive oil. Mix well and mash with wooden spoon. Add a few drops of vitamin E oil. Cover and shake. Put in a dark place and macerate for 6 weeks, shaking often. Strain well and pour into dark-coloured jar. Store at room temperature. To use, place 2–3 drops in ear canal 2–3 times a day.

IMPORTANT: Tea or infusions taken internally should be strained through a fine cloth or sieve before ingesting to remove tiny hairs, which can irritate the digestive tract. Some increase in coughing may occur when taken to treat respiratory problems; this is an indication phlegm is loosening and the herb is ultimately doing its job.

MUSTARD

Brassica nigra (Black Mustard)
Brassica alba (White Mustard)

FAMILY: *Brassicaceae*

OTHER NAMES: *Fr.* Moutarde

PARTS USED: Seeds, leaves, oil

CHARACTERISTICS: Warm, pungent

SYSTEMS AFFECTED: Lungs, stomach

ACTIONS: Rubifacient, irritant, stimulant, diuretic, emetic, carminative, tonic, diaphoretic

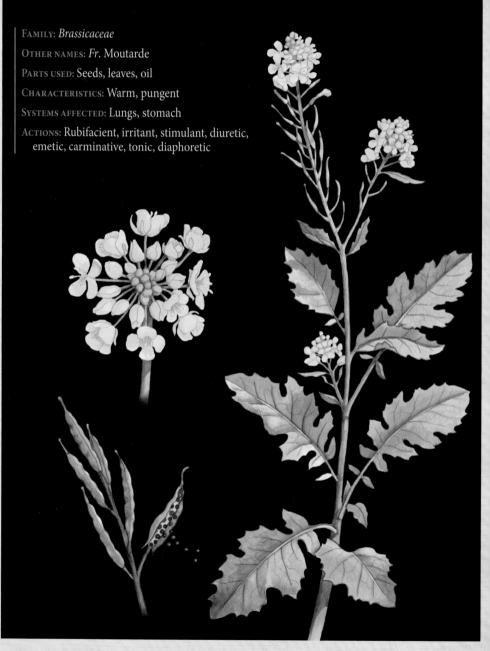

This common spice is a native plant of Europe, but is now often cultivated across North America, although it has escaped farms and is also growing wild just about everywhere. There are dozens of mustard species worldwide, and it is not only one of the oldest medicinal plants, but has also been used as a vegetable for hundreds of years. It is an erect annual that grows up to 1 metre in height. Its lower leaves are bristly and coarsely lobed, and the upper leaves are lance-shaped and hairless. The flowers of both Black and White Mustard species are yellow with 4 rounded petals arranged in the shape of a cross, Black being slightly smaller. The fruit of the two plants is quite different. The White variety grows horizontally and is hairy, roundish, and swollen, with 4–6 seeds, which are larger than the Black and have a sword-shaped beak at the tip. The short-beaked Black Mustard pod is smooth, erect, and flattened, with 10–12 small dark-red or black seeds. Black Mustard is stronger in flavour and pungency, and is more effective medicinally than the White variety. The young plants (before flowering) are nutritious, good in salads, and have a slightly pungent flavour.

MEDICINAL USES:

Chest congestion, arthritis, muscular or skeletal pain, athlete's foot

- Seeds and young leaves are a rich source of minerals and vitamins.
- Mustard plaster placed on the chest can relieve congestion in the lungs in pneumonia, pleurisy, or bronchitis by drawing blood from the site of inflammation to the surface. Also works for sinus infections, neuralgia, muscular or skeletal pain, and spasms.
- Bruised seeds mixed in warm water makes a nice footbath to help to get rid of a cold or dispel a headache. Soak for 10 minutes. Increases circulation.
- 1 tbsp. dry Mustard added to a cup of tepid water acts as an effective emetic. A teaspoon dissolved in boiling water will cure hiccups.
- In diluted form, the oil can be used as a liniment for aching muscles or arthritic joints, and is said to stimulate hair growth.
- A few drops of Mustard oil in a footbath can treat athlete's foot.
- Greens eaten raw or steamed can reduce cholesterol and provide magnesium and calcium, which are beneficial to menopausal women.
- Creates heat within the body, which can encourage sweating to cleanse toxins, and can stimulate healing when there is nerve damage.

MUSTARD PLASTER: Mix 1 tbsp. dry mustard with 1 tbsp. flour; mix in enough warm water to make a thick paste. Spread between two pieces of soft flannel, and place on chest until it becomes uncomfortably warm (approximately 10 minutes).

IMPORTANT: Not recommended for people with gastrointestinal ulcers or inflammatory kidney diseases. Never use the oil undiluted as it can cause blisters. Will cause vomiting in large doses.

OLD MAN'S BEARD

Usnea longissima
Usnea barbata

FAMILY: *Parmeliacaea*

OTHER NAMES: Usnea, Beard lichen

PARTS USED: Whole lichen

CHARACTERISTICS: Bitter, dry, cool

ACTIONS: Antibacterial, antiviral, anti-fungal, astringent, styptic, tonic, vulnerary

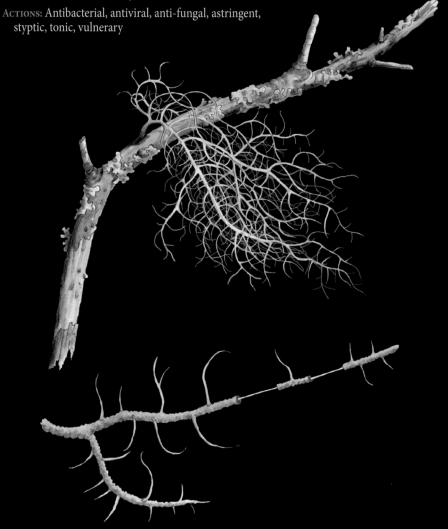

U snea or Old Man's Beard is a greenish-grey lichen, which is an organism that has a symbiotic relationship between algae and fungi. It grows on the branches of older trees, often ones that are sick or dying. It can be distinguished from other similar-looking lichens by a white elastic thread (fungus) running through the herb that is revealed by gently pulling apart a filament (algae). There are hundreds of species, and it has been used for centuries worldwide as a powerful anti-microbial that is effective against a wide range of pathogens. It can grow up to 20 cm. long, and since it is very slow growing, it should be harvested from dead or fallen branches to avoid over-harvesting. Choose a clean location as it easily absorbs heavy metals and pollution from the environment. Store in a dry place.

MEDICINAL USES:

Bacterial, viral, and fungal infections, wounds

- Used on a wide range of diseases; as it can kill pathogens without disrupting most gut flora, it is a valuable treatment for many infections, both viral and bacterial. Effective against Gram-positive bacteria like streptococcus and staphylococcus, as well as pneumonia, upper-respiratory tract infections, and urinary tract infections, but unlike most antibiotics, it won't disrupt healthy gut flora. Combats common viral infections such as herpes and Epstein–Barr. It works through the mucous membranes to fight lung and bronchial infections with yellow or green phlegm, and fevers.
- Effective both topically and internally against fungal infections like candida, athlete's foot, and ringworm, although lifestyle and diet modifications should be made in order to completely eradicate the infections, as they are usually hard to get rid of.
- Heals wounds, bites, and stings, and can help prevent infection.
- May be useful in treatment for gastric ulcers.
- Indigenous peoples in North America consider Old Man's Beard to have a sacred relationship with the trees, helping them fight off infection.

TINCTURE: Place ¼ cup chopped fresh or dried herb into a pot with ½ cup water. Bring to a boil, cover, and simmer 15–20 minutes until reduced to ⅓ cup. Cool for a few minutes and pour into a small Mason jar. Add ⅓ cup vodka and mix well. Screw on lid and let sit for 2 weeks, shaking daily to mix. Strain mixture and transfer to an amber tincture bottle. Take 6–12 drops 3 times a day.

IMPORTANT: Avoid during pregnancy. May irritate the digestive system in large amounts.

PINEAPPLE WEED

Matricaria discoida (matricarioides)

FAMILY: *Asteraceae*

OTHER NAMES: Wild Camomile, Rayless Mayweed, Disc Mayweed

PARTS USED: Flowers

CHARACTERISTICS: Aromatic, bitter, neutral, spicy

SYSTEMS AFFECTED: Liver, stomach

ACTIONS: Antiseptic, carminative, diaphoretic, sedative, antispasmodic, analgesic, anthelmintic

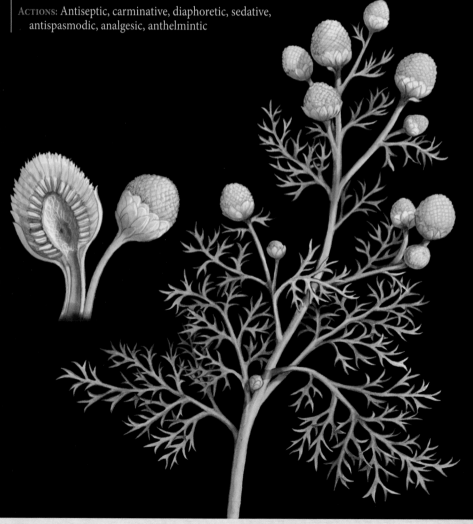

This annual plant resembles Camomile but without the petals, and is distinguished by its scent, which lies somewhere between Chamomile and pineapple. Its erect stem has many finely dissected leaves, and usually grows to about 30 cm. high. The solitary, terminal, cone-shaped flowerheads are greenish-yellow and encircled by bracts. This plant grows in disturbed areas, roadsides, and pathways from June until early fall. Collect the flowers early in the summer and dry for later use.

MEDICINAL USES:

Insomnia, digestive problems, skin disorders, fevers

- Infusion of flowers is effective for relieving indigestion, bloating, and constipation.
- Calming and sedative, it relieves insomnia and reduces anxiety.
- Stimulates milk production in nursing women.
- Induces sweating to reduce fevers; good for colds and flu.
- Flowerheads are packed with nutrients, which give an energetic boost.
- Helps expel intestinal worms.
- Works externally as a mouthwash and gargle, and as a compress or bath preparation for insect bites and skin disorders such as psoriasis and eczema. Reduces inflammation and relieves pain.
- Indigenous peoples used it for treating stomach problems, gas, sores, fevers and menstrual pain.

OTHER USES:
- Indigenous peoples use these aromatic flowers as perfume, often carrying them in medicine pouches along with Sweetgrass and Cedar or Fir. The dried plants have also been used to line cradles and stuff pillows.
- Makes an effective insect repellent.

INFUSION: Mix 1 tbsp. young flowerheads in 1 cup boiling water; steep 5–10 minutes. Drink 2–3 times a day.

IMPORTANT: In large quantities this herb may cause stomach upset or diarrhea. People with sensitive skin or allergies may experience inflammation or itching.

PITCHER PLANT

Sarracenia purpurea

FAMILY: *Sarraceniaceae*

OTHER NAMES: Eve's Cups, Flycatcher, Fly-trap, Water Cup, *Fr.* Népenthès, Oreille de cochon, Petits cochons

PARTS USED: Roots, leaves

CHARACTERISTICS: Bitter

SYSTEMS AFFECTED: Lungs, liver, stomach, kidney, uterus

ACTIONS: Diuretic, hepatic, stimulating tonic, laxative, stomachic, astringent (root)

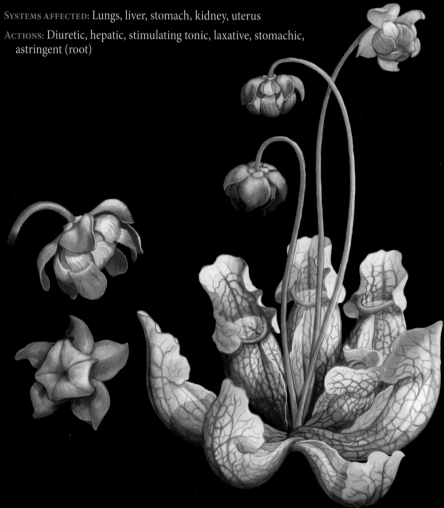

This strange and unique carnivorous perennial is native to North America, and can be found in bogs and wet meadows throughout eastern Canada. Its leaves are evergreen, usually 15–23 cm., reddish to green, veined, and shaped like an inflated tube topped by an arching hood. The single purple nodding flower, which blooms from May to July, grows atop a scape of 30–60 cm. high. The leaves fill with rainwater and trap insects and other small creatures inside, due to the downward-pointing hairs inside the tube. It then releases enzymes that digest the insect, from which it obtains most of its nutrients.

MEDICINAL USES:

Fevers, constipation, indigestion, kidney ailments

- Dried leaf tea used to ease fevers and chills.
- Root used to reduce sluggishness, create movement. Laxative, stimulates a sluggish liver, relieves stomach upset.
- Relieves kidney, urinary tract, and bladder infections.
- Infusion of dried leaves used to facilitate childbirth, expel the placenta, and prevent sickness after childbirth; brings on menstruation in cases of amenorrhea.
- Cold decoction of leaves and root used in treatment of whooping cough.
- An infusion of the roots was once used as a remedy and prevention for smallpox by North American Indigenous peoples. It is highly regarded by the Cree and often added to other medicines to increase effectiveness.
- An extract made from the plant, called Sarapin, can be injected as an alternative to steroids or cortisone to relieve pain, although it is rarely used in medical practice, perhaps due to the fact it cannot be patented.

IMPORTANT: Do not use if pregnant or breastfeeding.

PLANTAIN

Plantago major (Common Plantain)
Plantago lanceolata (English Plantain)

FAMILY: *Plantaginaceae*

OTHER NAMES: Englishman's Foot, Ribwort, *Fr.* Plantain

PARTS USED: Leaves and seeds

CHARACTERISTICS: Bland, slightly bitter, cool, drying

SYSTEMS AFFECTED: Bladder, small intestine, gallbladder

ACTIONS: Diuretic, alterative, anti-inflammatory, mild laxative, astringent, anti-microbial, antiseptic, hemostatic

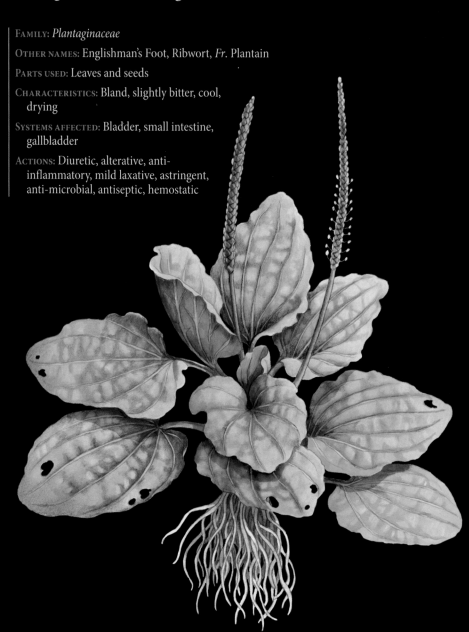

One of the most common herbs found in the Maritimes, Common Plantain (*P. major*) grows on practically every lawn, roadside, or abandoned lot. It will pop up virtually anywhere, including paved driveways or in sidewalk cracks, and needs very little sun. It grows close to the ground, with a rosette of ovate, blunt leaves 10–25 cm. long, with long fibrous ribs. The erect flower spikes are dark green and can be up to 30 cm. long. The narrow-leaved English Plantain (*P. lanceolata*) has longer-stemmed flower spikes, but many of the same medicinal properties as the common variety. The young plants of both varieties may be eaten fresh in salads if harvested in the spring. To preserve for later, they should be gathered during flowering throughout the summer and dried quickly, as they tend to discolour rapidly. Use only plants from yards that have never been sprayed with chemicals.

MEDICINAL USES:

Wounds, insect bites, urinary tract infections, digestive tract inflammation

- Bruised leaves may be applied directly to stings or insect bites, or used in a salve or ointment, as it soothes and relieves pain and itching.
- Astringent, it stops bleeding, promotes healing of exterior wounds, and is rich in tannin, which helps draw tissues together.
- Helps heal urinary tract infections and other internal inflammation, including hepatitis.
- Tea brewed from leaves and seeds, which are high in mucilage, is a folk remedy for diarrhea, dysentery, and bleeding hemorrhoids. Some studies indicate the leaves and seeds may also reduce blood pressure and lower cholesterol.
- Infusion of the leaves can be used as a gentle expectorant, to soothe an irritated throat, or to ease gastric inflammation and bleeding mucous membranes.
- Leaves are high in calcium and vitamins A, C, and K. Combines well with Calendula, Yarrow, Chamomile, and Agrimony in infusions.
- Leaves may be heated in warm water and applied to swollen joints or sore muscles to relieve pain.

OTHER USES AND FOLKLORE:
- Cold tea used as a hair rinse for dandruff.
- Once believed to cure rabies and ward off snakes.
- Put on aching feet after a long trek to relieve soreness and fatigue.

HEALING SALVE: Place 2 cups of entire chopped Plantain plant in a non-metallic pan, add ½ cup lard or coconut oil, heat slowly on low heat until mixture becomes green and wilted; strain, pour into jars, and cool. Will harden slightly; good for use on burns, rashes, bites, and other sores.

POND LILY

Nymphaea odorata (Water Lily)
Nuphar variegate (Cow Lily)

FAMILY: *Nymphaeaceae*

OTHER NAMES: Water Lily, Beaver Root, *Fr.* Nénuphar

PARTS USED: Rhizome, flowers, stems

CHARACTERISTICS: Bitter, cool

SYSTEMS AFFECTED: Nervous, intestinal, heart

ACTIONS: Anaphrodisiac, astringent, demulcent, cardiotonic, antispasmodic, antiscrophulactic, anodyne, sedative

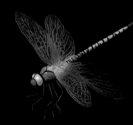

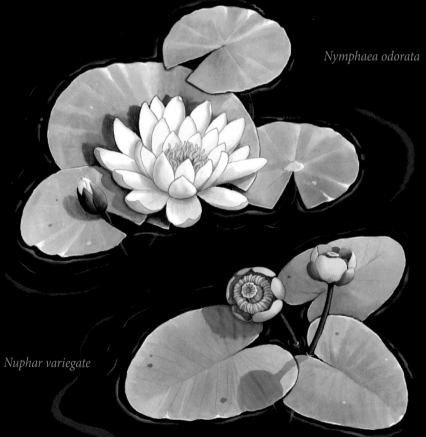

Nymphaea odorata

Nuphar variegate

Water or Pond Lily is a native perennial aquatic plant that grows from an anchor of rootlets buried in the mud of a pond or lake. Its long stem extends upward to the surface, where its flat, waxy, orbicular leaves—dark green on top, purplish underneath and notched at the base—float on the surface. The large, sweetly scented flowers of the Water variety (*N. odorata*) float on the surface, and are around 12 cm. in diameter and bowl-shaped with many petals. They can be white or pinkish with a yellow centre, and they close up in the evening. The Yellow Pond Lily or Cow Lily (*N. variegata*) has similar properties but is less effective medicinally than *Nymphaea*. The roots can be harvested in the fall when the flowers have died down, and may be dried and ground for later use.

MEDICINAL USES:

Diarrhea, chronic bronchitis, leukorrhea, skin inflammation, boils, mouth infections

- Mi'kmaq use the mashed root as a poultice for sore limbs, arthritis, and as a food source.
- A tea made from Water Lily roots contains tannin and mucilage, and was once used to treat tuberculosis and chronic bronchitis, as well as diarrhea and other gastrointestinal inflammation. It can also be used as a douche to treat vaginal discharge (leukorrhea).
- The flowers are reported to reduce libido and have a tranquilizing effect, reduce pain and anxiety, and help relieve insomnia. Some claim that smoking the dried buds has a psychoactive effect.
- A poultice of the mashed root is used in the treatment of swellings, boils, wounds, bee stings, and inflamed tissues, and when mixed with lemon juice may reduce the appearance of pimples and freckles,
- Infusion may be used as a mouthwash to treat inflamed gums and sore throat.

OTHER USES: Flower buds can be cooked as a vegetable; ripe seeds may be ground into meal and used as a flour substitute.

INFUSION: Mix 1–2 tsp. dried root in 1 cup boiling water; steep 10 minutes. Strain, take 2 times a day.

FOLKLORE: The scientific name derives from the Greek word "numphe," or "water nymph," and is associated with purity, chastity, or virginity—no doubt due to its anaphrodisiac properties. The Lotus, also a member of the Water Lily family, has been used as a symbol of the Buddha and immortality for thousands of years.

IMPORTANT: Avoid use during pregnancy or breastfeeding. May interfere with drugs affecting the central nervous system (opioids, antidepressants, antipsychotics). Do not consume more than the recommended dose, as it is potentially toxic.

PURPLE LOOSESTRIFE

Lythrum salicaria

FAMILY: *Lythraceae*

OTHER NAMES: Rainbowweed, Purple Willow Herb, Flowering Sally, *Fr.* Salicaire commune

PARTS USED: Aerial

CHARACTERISTICS: Sour, cool, dry, moist

ACTIONS: Astringent (leaves and stems), mucilaginous (flowering spikes), antibacterial, antioxidant, antispasmodic, diuretic, demulcent, anti-inflammatory, styptic, tonic, vulnerary

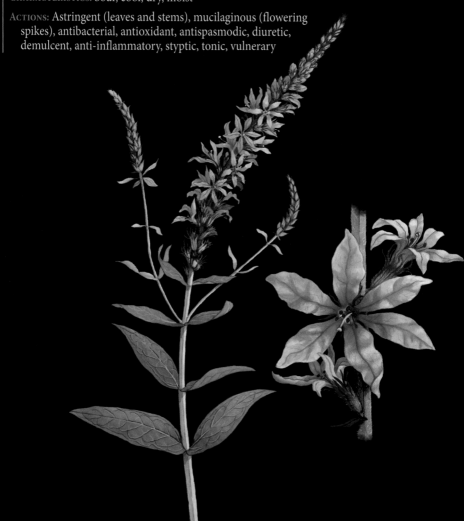

Purple Loosestrife has a bad reputation for being an invasive species, although it really only invades areas that have been laid fallow by human intervention; it usually remains under control in a natural habitat. It is a handsome perennial, growing up to 2.5 metres high, with square or many-sided stems branching towards the top. The leaves are lance-shaped, attach closely to the stem, and are usually opposite. The taproots are woody with a creeping rhizome. The bright purplish or crimson flowers grow along the top part of the spike from the bottom up, in whorls of 6 or 8 flowers, each one composed of a tube with (usually) 6 equal petals and 12 stamens. They produce up to 3 million seeds a year and also reproduce from the rhizomes, so it can spread rapidly, choking out other native plants. It grows mainly in wet, swampy areas, with flowers blooming from July to September. Gather when in full bloom and dry in the shade, storing in cloth bags for later use.

MEDICINAL USES:

Chronic diarrhea, leukorrhea, sore dry eyes, fevers, skin inflammation, and sores

- Valuable healing plant as it contains a balance of astringent (tightens and restores tone to tissues) and mucilage (soothes, lubricates, and eases inflammation). Excellent for chronic diarrhea, dysentery, enteritis, IBS, and leaky gut, as it repairs tissues and reduces pain and inflammation. Strangely enough, it also works well for constipation as it tones the mucus membranes and strengthens the intestinal walls, improving motility.
- A sterile infusion makes an excellent eyewash for sore, dry eyes.
- Decoction used to bring down fevers and to treat liver problems.
- For external applications to sores, ulcers, bruises, abrasions, irritations, and to stop bleeding, prepare a strong decoction and apply as an ointment or poultice.
- Stems may be chewed to prevent bleeding gums; a decoction of leaves and stems may also be used as a mouthwash for irritated gums or throat.
- Decoction used as a douche for leukorrhea, or may be applied to hemorrhoids.
- Was once a valuable treatment for cholera, drunk in small doses of warm tea mixed with Ginger.

OTHER USES AND FOLKLORE:
- Ancient Greeks hung garlands of Purple Loosestrife around the necks of oxen, as they believed it helped them to work better as a team.
- Once used as a hair dye and to drive away insects.
- A decoction may be used to soak wood or rope to prevent rotting.

DECOCTION: Place 1–2 tsp. dried herb in 1 cup of hot water; steep 1 hour. Take 1–3 cups per day.

PURSLANE

Portulaca oleracea

FAMILY: *Portulacaceae*

OTHER NAMES: Pigweed, Little Hogweed, *Fr.* Pourpier

PARTS USED: Aerial

CHARACTERISTICS: Cooling, slightly sour, salty

SYSTEMS AFFECTED: Liver, stomach

ACTIONS: Antioxidant, anti-inflammatory, anti-fungal, diuretic, vermicide

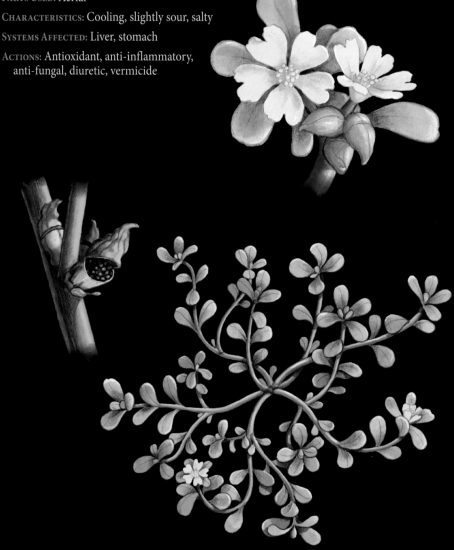

One of the most nutritious wild greens available, Purslane is largely ignored in North America and pulled out as a weed, but is considered a delicacy in many other countries. Probably originating in Asia or Africa, it is now found throughout the world, and is very high in omega-3 fatty acids, antioxidants, vitamins A, B, C, and E, and beta-carotene, as well as fibre, potassium, and magnesium. Its round red stems and thick, succulent, spatula-shaped, dark-green leaves creep along the ground in waste places and in gardens. The tiny yellow flowers have 4–6 petals, and grow in the leaf rosettes. Best if picked in July, before flowering.

MEDICINAL USES:

High blood pressure, diarrhea, skin inflammation, coughs, gum irritation

- Very nutritious; contains vitamins A, B, C, and E, as well as potassium, magnesium, and calcium. Can be eaten raw in salads or added to soups and stews.
- Contains high levels of omega-3 fatty acids, which improve heart health and reduce blood pressure and risk of cardiovascular disease. The presence of fibre helps in weight reduction, and the minerals may help prevent osteoporosis and improve circulation.
- Contains mucilage, which is soothing and cooling. In a small clinical trial, oral ingestion showed improvements in pulmonary function of patients with asthma. Honey added to the juice makes a syrup that is effective in relieving dry coughs.
- Stops hemorrhaging and reduces uterine bleeding.
- Treats diarrhea, intestinal bleeding, and hemorrhoids.
- High in antioxidants, which eliminate free radicals and may prevent certain cancers.
- Juice applied directly to the skin can relieve pain from bee stings and burns, reduce wrinkles, and remove blemishes.
- Beta-carotene helps improve vision and prevents eye degeneration as we age. Poultices of the juice may be applied to the eyes to reduce redness.
- Seeds were once crushed and boiled in wine to give to children as a vermifuge.
- Juice, when mixed with a drop of oil of roses, soothes inflamed gums and helps fasten loose teeth.

OTHER USES AND FOLKLORE: Was once strewn around the bed to ward off evil spirits.

IMPORTANT: Not recommended if you have kidney stones, due to the plant's relatively high content of oxalic acid.

QUEEN ANNE'S LACE

Daucus carota

FAMILY: *Apiaceae*

OTHER NAMES: Wild carrot, Bee's Nest, Bird's Nest, *Fr.* Carotte sauvage

PARTS USED: Root, leaves, and seeds

CHARACTERISTICS: Bitter

SYSTEMS AFFECTED: Bladder, kidney, uterus

ACTIONS: Diuretic, purgative, vermifuge, anthelmintic, carminative, antilithic, emmenagogue

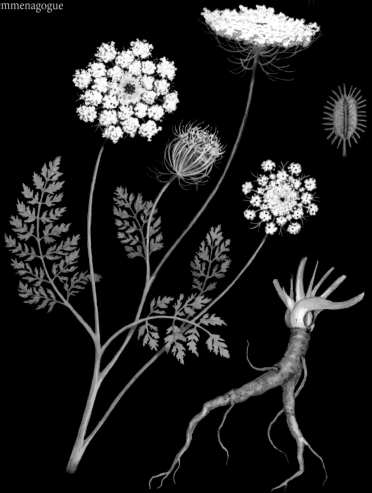

This biennial herb is found along roadsides and fields throughout most of Canada during the summer months, and is a direct descendent of the garden-variety carrot. A native of southern Europe, its stems are up to 0.9 metres high, and are erect and branched with finely dissected, fern-like leaves. Flowers are densely clustered white umbels radiating from the central stalk with a tiny purple or pink flower in the centre. As the seeds ripen, the umbels contract and curve inwards, forming a nest-like appearance, hence the name Bird's Nest. The large taproot is whitish and bitter and smells like carrot. It is harvested in late summer and should be cut longitudinally and dried, or the tender smaller roots may be eaten fresh in the spring. The leaves should be picked in July before it has gone to seed; the seeds are more potent when collected just before they are fully mature.

MEDICINAL USES:

Urinary antiseptic, kidney stones, gout, rheumatism, flatulence and colic, diuretic for edema

- An infusion of the leaves is effective in the treatment of digestive disorders, as it soothes the digestive tract and relieves gas. A wonderful cleansing herb, it can relieve chronic kidney problems, gout, stones, and bladder infections. Diuretic, it is useful in treating edema and in weight loss to eliminate water retention.
- The seeds are known to stimulate the pituitary gland, which in turn stimulates sex hormones to bring on menstruation. It has been used to prevent conception, although when use is stopped, it may increase chances of conceiving, as it tones the uterus. Reduces heavy flow and helps with the symptoms of endometriosis.
- The root is slightly bitter but edible, and is rich in vitamin A. It can be used in a poultice to ease the pain of skin ulcers, or in infusions as a mild laxative, diuretic, or to expel kidney stones.
- The Mi'kmaq have used it as a purgative, and it has been used widely for lack of appetite, to expel intestinal worms, and as a poultice to reduce swelling and soothe sores.

OTHER USES: Seeds contain an essential oil that is used in anti-wrinkle cream, and a decoction of the seeds and root makes a good insecticide. The seeds can also be used as flavouring for soups and stews.

FOLKLORE: The tiny red flower in the centre is apparently how Queen Anne's Lace got its name, since Queen Anne, according to legend, pricked her finger while making lace, leaving one droplet of blood. The flower was once believed to cure epilepsy.

INFUSION: Pour 1 cup of boiling water onto 1 tsp. of dried leaves or bruised seeds; infuse 10–15 minutes. Drink 3 times a day.

TINCTURE: Use 20 drops twice a day.

IMPORTANT: Should not be used by pregnant women, as it may stimulate contractions.

RASPBERRY

Rubus idaeus

FAMILY: *Rosaceae*

OTHER NAMES: *Fr.* Framboise

PARTS USED: Leaf, fruit, root

CHARACTERISTICS: Mild, bitter, cool

SYSTEMS AFFECTED: Spleen, liver, kidneys, reproductive organs

ACTIONS: Astringent, anti-inflammatory, hemostatic, alterative, parturient, anti-emetic

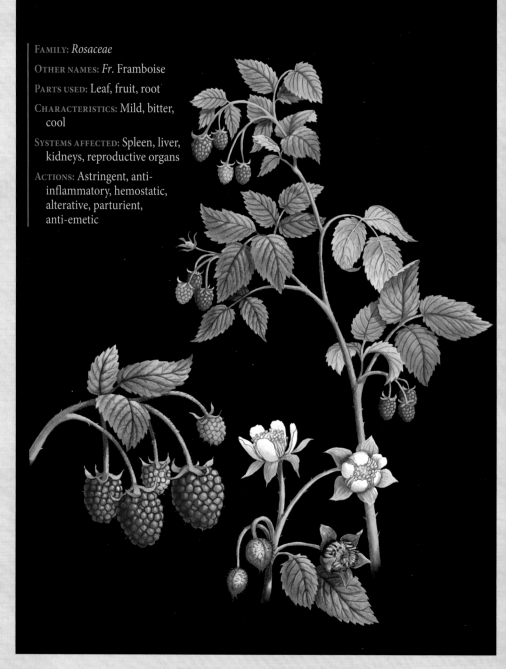

The sweet red fruit of the Raspberry plant is well known to most North Americans, but few know of the plant's use as an herbal remedy. A relative of the Rose family, Raspberry has creeping perennial roots and grows up to 1.8 metres high. It's easily identified by its tangle of bristly vines along roadsides and fields. Its compound leaves are alternate and pointed, with 3 to 7 toothed leaflets. The small white or pinkish 5-petalled flowers bloom in June or July, and are followed by clusters of bright red berries, which usually appear in August. The leaves should be harvested on a dry day in early summer and dried quickly to prevent mould from forming on the leaves.

MEDICINAL USES

Helps birthing process, fevers, diarrhea, colds, incontinence, menorrhagia, sore throat

- Berries are high in vitamin B and C as well as magnesium, potassium, iron, and calcium, so they work well for immune support, as well as to keep women healthy by balancing hormones and strengthening the wall of the uterus.
- A wonderful uterine tonic, the leaf tea has been used for centuries by women to strengthen the muscles of the uterus, facilitate delivery, prevent miscarriage, and reduce excessive menstrual bleeding. It tones the uterus after delivery and has been used to treat fibroids, endometriosis, and heavy, painful, or irregular periods.
- Reduces fevers, sore throat, cold symptoms, and diarrhea.
- Nourishes the blood; replenishes iron and other minerals.
- Leaves are crushed and used in an infusion by the Mi'kmaq to relieve stomach upset and prevent vomiting. Roots are used to treat diarrhea, and bark tea relieves stomachaches.
- Applied topically to wounds, a leaf poultice speeds the healing process and prevents infection. A strong tea can soothe sunburn, eczema, and rashes, and when used as a mouthwash, it can improve symptoms of gingivitis.

INFUSION: Mix small handful of fresh or dried leaves in 2 cups of water; simmer for a few minutes. Cool for 15 minutes, strain, and drink two or three times a day.

IMPORTANT: Not suitable for people with gastritis or peptic ulcer, since it contains tannin. Pregnant women should avoid using until the last 2 months of pregnancy.

RED CLOVER

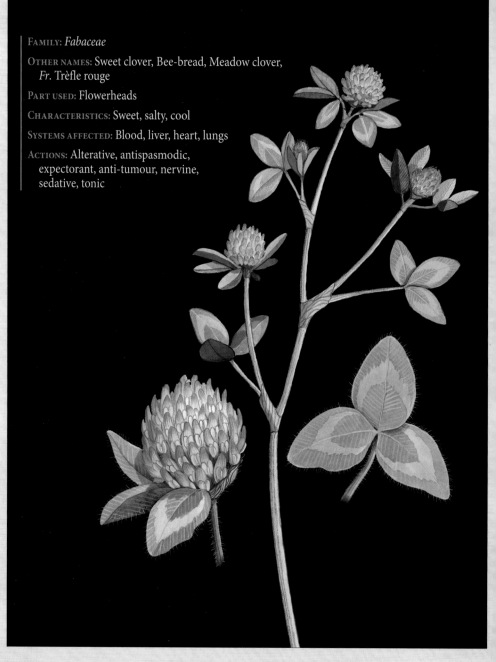

Trifolium pratense

FAMILY: *Fabaceae*

OTHER NAMES: Sweet clover, Bee-bread, Meadow clover,
Fr. Trèfle rouge

PART USED: Flowerheads

CHARACTERISTICS: Sweet, salty, cool

SYSTEMS AFFECTED: Blood, liver, heart, lungs

ACTIONS: Alterative, antispasmodic,
expectorant, anti-tumour, nervine,
sedative, tonic

Fields of Red Clover may be seen across the Maritimes in the summer, its sweet scent permeating the air. It is often planted by farmers as a cover crop to improve the nitrogen levels in the soil, protect from erosion, and provide feed for animals, but grows wild almost everywhere. It is a short-lived perennial, with several stems from 30 to 60 cm. high, arising from the one root and three oval leaflets with a "V" marked in a lighter green. The flowers are pink or red in a round dense terminal, and bloom from June to September. Originally from Europe, Asia, and Africa, Red Clover has been used as a medicinal remedy for centuries. Pick the flowerheads in early summer and dry for later use.

MEDICINAL USES:

Blood thinner, skin diseases, congestion, fevers, menopause, coughs

- Blood purifier and blood thinner, it may be beneficial for those with thrombosis or thick blood where clots may form. (However, it should not be used if you are on blood-thinning medication.) A combination of Red Clover and Burdock Root is considered an excellent blood tonic.
- Increases elasticity of arteries, and may lower levels of LDL cholesterol, reducing the risk of cardiovascular disease, especially after menopause.
- A rich source of isoflavones, it can mimic estrogen, relieving hot flashes and other discomforts of menopause, as well as symptoms of PMS. Helps prevent bone loss and may improve healing of broken bones.
- Used in salves and liniments for skin complaints, especially in children. Good for eruptions, psoriasis, eczema, bee stings, etc. (However, it should not be used on open wounds.)
- Some Mi'kmaq use the blossoms steeped as a tea to bring down fever, or in a poultice for sore eyes, burns, and stings.
- Effective for coughs, colds, mucous congestion, asthma, and bronchitis; the flowers were once dried and smoked to relieve asthma. Once used as a remedy for whooping cough.
- Regulates digestion, improves appetite, and increases the detoxification ability of the liver.
- Contains several compounds that have anti-cancer properties, and although little clinical research has been done to prove its effectiveness, Red Clover appears to limit the growth of cancer by preventing the growth of new blood vessels that feed the tumour. It is used in the Hoxsey Herbal Therapy anti-cancer formula, and is sometimes included in some forms of Essiac tea.

INFUSION: Pour 1 cup of boiling water onto 1–3 tsp. dried flowers. Infuse 10–15 minutes. Take 3 times a day.

IMPORTANT: Women with hormone-related conditions such as endometriosis, uterine fibroids, and/or breast, ovarian, or uterine cancers should avoid taking Red Clover due to the presence of phytoestrogens.

SARSAPARILLA

Aralia nudicaulis (Wild)
Aralia racemosa (Spikenard)

FAMILY: *Araliaceae*

OTHER NAMES: False Sarsaparilla, Small Spikenard, Wild Liquorice, Rabbit Root, *Fr.* Salsepareille Sauvage

PARTS USED: Root, berries

CHARACTERISTICS: Sweet, pungent, aromatic

SYSTEMS AFFECTED: Lungs, stomach

ACTIONS: Alterative, diaphoretic, diuretic, pectoral, stimulant

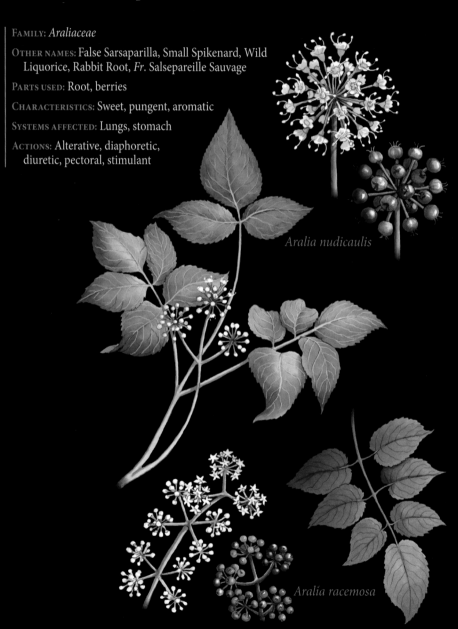

Aralia nudicaulis

Aralia racemosa

*A*ralia nudicaulis, or Wild Sarsaparilla, has been widely used by Indigenous peoples across North America for centuries, and as a substitute in formulas for the unrelated tropical variety, *Smilax ornata*. It is a perennial of the Ginseng family that grows to a height of 60 cm. with cord-like runners. The stems are smooth and grow out of the runners, dividing into 3 branches, each producing large, finely toothed compound leaves composed of usually 5 leaflets. The leaves are often reddish early in the spring and turn green as the plant matures. Usually, 3 globe-shaped clusters of tiny white flowers will appear on scapes the same height as the stems in June or July, and are followed by edible black berries that taste spicy and sweet. *Aralia racemosa*, or Spikenard, is quite a bit taller, often growing as high as 1.5 metres. Its leaves are more heart-shaped and the flowers grow in many clusters along the stem. Both varieties prefer moist, shady woods, and are used for similar purposes. The rootstock, which has a sweet–spicy taste, is best collected in the fall and dried for later use.

MEDICINAL USES:

Pulmonary diseases, fevers, skin problems, rheumatism

The Mi'kmaq have a wide variety of uses for Sarsaparilla:
- The boiled rhizome can be mashed and used as a poultice for wounds, sores, burns, itchy skin, ulcers, eczema, and rheumatism.
- The dried and ground rhizomes of Sarsaparilla and Sweet Flag can be steeped in water and administered as cough medicine.
- Decoction from the powdered rhizome encourages sweating and is good for ridding the body of colds and flu. Its anti-inflammatory properties make it good for chronic bronchial and renal infections that are difficult to get rid of. It has also been found useful as a wash for treating shingles.
- Tonic for stress, it nourishes and relaxes the adrenal glands. Best used long term.
- Fresh mashed roots can be used to treat sores, draw out infection, and stem nosebleeds.

OTHER USES:
- Rootstock has been used as a substitute for the tropical medicinal herb Sarsaparilla (*Smilax ornata*).
- Used as flavouring for root beer.
- Since the root is highly nutritious, it was often mixed with oil and used by Indigenous peoples as an emergency food.
- Makes a pleasant herbal tea by boiling in water until it turns reddish-brown.
- Jelly or wine can be made from the fruit.

SHEEP SORREL

Rumex acetosella

FAMILY: *Polygonaceae*

OTHER NAMES: Garden sorrel, Sourweed, Red sorrel, Field sorrel, Spinach dock, *Fr.* Oseille

PARTS USED: Leaves, root, seeds

CHARACTERISTICS: Cool, dry, sour

ACTIONS: Mildly antiseptic, laxative, diuretic, antiscorbutic, febrifuge

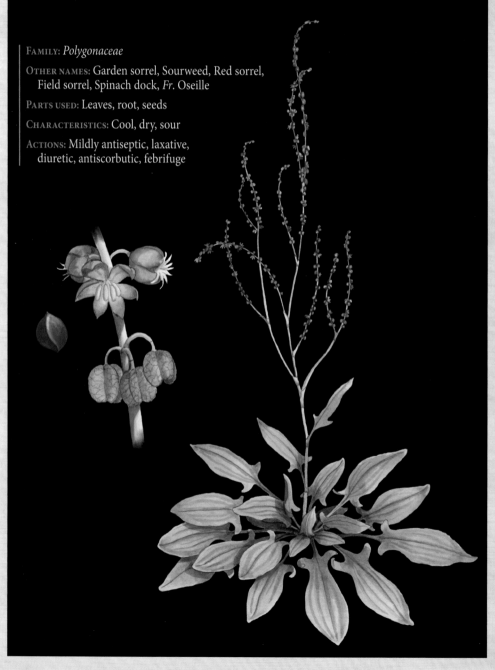

This common perennial originating from Europe grows abundantly in meadows and pastures throughout Canada and has been used around the world for centuries in salads, as a vegetable, and as a potherb. It has a sharp, tangy taste due to the presence of oxalic acid, and is loaded with nutrients, including vitamins A and C, iron, magnesium, potassium, and calcium. Often up to 60 cm. high, it branches at the top, and its leaves are shaped like an arrowhead. The dark red or purplish flower spikes stand out in a field of grasses. Its flowers turn into reddish-brown seedpods in the fall. Leaves are best harvested early in the summer when they are tender.

MEDICINAL USES:

Fevers, inflammation, cancer, sinusitis, Type 2 diabetes, hemorrhoids, skin irritations

- Leaves can be eaten raw in mixed salads or cooked in stews, much like spinach. Perfectly safe in moderate quantities, but due to the presence of oxalic acid, should not be consumed in excessive amounts raw. If cooking a large potful, change the water halfway through the process to remove the oxalic acid. Use only a stainless steel or glass pot, as other materials may affect the taste.
- Infusion used as a diuretic and appetite stimulant, for treating kidney stones, and to reduce fever and soothe an upset stomach.
- The root and seed were once used as an astringent to stop hemorrhage.
- The juice from the leaves is used as a gargle for mouth ulcers, in a compress to treat cysts and itching, heal wounds, staunch bleeding, and reduce swelling and inflammation. It makes a cooling drink for fevers.
- Improves digestion and provides nutrients and antioxidants, which may help prevent certain cancers, lower blood pressure, and improve the condition of diabetics. It is a key ingredient in the formula for Essiac tea.

OTHER USES: Roots and stems are used to obtain dyes; the juice is sometimes used to remove stains from linen.

IMPORTANT: Since the presence of oxalic acid is quite high, do not consume in large quantities.

SILVERWEED

Argentina anserina

FAMILY: *Rosaceae*

OTHER NAMES: Argentine, Crampweed, Goosewort, Moon Grass, Trailing Tansy, Silvery Cinquefoil, *Fr.* Potentille des oies, Argentine

PARTS USED: Root, herb, dried

CHARACTERISTICS: Bitter, sweet, cooling

SYSTEMS AFFECTED: Digestive system

ACTIONS: Astringent, anti-catarrhal, diuretic, anti-inflammatory, antispasmodic, hemostatic, tonic

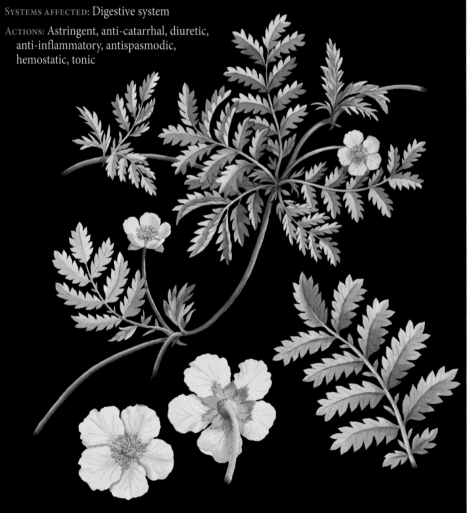

This ground-hugging native perennial usually grows to a height of only 20–40 cm. in the wild, but has red-coloured runners that can reach up to 1.8 metres long. Each tuft of leaves arising from the runners produces 1 yellow 5-petalled flower on a leafless stalk. They bloom between June and August and close at night and on cloudy days. The compound leaves are pinnately divided into up to 20 toothed leaflets, some smaller ones mixed in with the larger ones. They are hairy and either green or silver on the top, and woolly and silver underneath. Silverweed grows in ditches and roadsides as well as fields and is a favourite snack of geese, hence the name "Goosewort." The roots can be harvested late in the summer or fall and dried; the leaves should be picked in early summer and dried in the shade.

MEDICINAL USES:

Coughs, hemorrhoids, diarrhea, gingivitis

- Mild astringent, especially the roots, with a gentle action on the gastrointestinal tract. Antispasmodic, it checks bleeding hemorrhoids and treats diarrhea when accompanied by indigestion.
- Good for a cough with thick yellow phlegm, it reduces mucus production, cools inflammation.
- Strong infusion has a lot of tannin and is used as a gargle for sore throat, and a mouthwash for sore gums and gingivitis.
- Eases menstrual cramps and excessive menstrual bleeding.
- Rootstock may be dried and ground to a powder for use in salves, compresses, or bath preparations. Used as a local analgesic and anti-inflammatory to treat hemorrhoids, swelling, burns, and skin ailments. Bruised leaves may be applied directly on the skin for the same purpose.

OTHER USES:
- The root was used for centuries by some Indigenous peoples as a nutritious food when no other food was available. It can be eaten raw, boiled, or roasted, and has a nutty and somewhat starchy flavour. The leaves may also be eaten raw or cooked.
- A leaf placed in the shoe can prevent blisters and sweaty feet.
- An infusion was once said to remove freckles.

INFUSION: Mix ½–1 tsp. of dried herb in 1 cup boiling water; steep 10 minutes. Drink 2–3 times per day.

SKULLCAP

Scutellaria lateriflora (Blue Skullcap)
Scutellaria galericulata (Marsh Skullcap)

FAMILY: *Lamiaceae*

OTHER NAMES: Blue Skullcap, Mad-dog Skullcap,
Virginia Skullcap, Madweed, Helmetflower,
Marsh Skullcap (*S. galericulata*) *Fr.* Scutellaire

PARTS USED: Aerial

CHARACTERISTICS: Bitter, cold, drying

SYSTEMS AFFECTED: Nervous system, uterus,
heart

ACTIONS: Sedative, anti-inflammatory,
antioxidant, nervine, tonic, antispasmodic,
emmenagogue, febrifuge

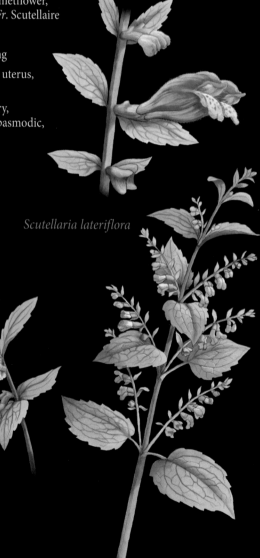

Scutellaria lateriflora

Scutellaria galericulata

A perennial plant that is native to North America, Skullcap has been used by Indigenous peoples for centuries to treat nervous disorders and menstrual problems. The plant prefers partially shaded wetland areas, its erect, square stem growing to a height of 45–60 cm. with occasional branches. It has broad, lance-shaped, toothed leaves in opposite pairs, and from July to September it bears blue–lavender, 2-lipped, tube-shaped flowers; the upper lip forming a hood, the lower lip having 2 lobes, somewhat resembling a helmet or cap. It is easily identified by a protuberance on the upper calyx. It should not be confused with the Chinese variety (*Scutellaria baicalensis* or Huang qin), which has different medicinal properties. Skullcap should be harvested in summertime while the flowers are in full bloom, and dried for future use (although they are best used fresh in making tinctures if possible).

MEDICINAL USES:

Nervous disorders, insomnia, epilepsy, suppressed menstruation

- Tonic and restorative properties help nourish the nervous system, it relaxes nervous tension during prolonged periods of stress; calms, promotes sleep; eases anxiety, busy mind, panic attacks. Effects are cumulative and it may be used over long periods of time. Not a strong sedative but may be combined with other herbs like Valerian for sleep.
- Eases PMS symptoms, promotes menstruation. Some Indigenous peoples have used it in traditional ceremonies to bring young girls to womanhood.
- Contains scutellarin, a flavonoid with antispasmodic properties, so it can be used to treat epilepsy, convulsions, and spasms.
- Helps with alcohol and drug withdrawal; lessens the severity of symptoms and detoxifies.
- Eases the symptoms of neuralgia and fibromyalgia; used in cases of lupus to reduce spasms without stimulating the immune system.
- Relieves incessant coughing and pneumonia.
- Reduces fever, increases blood flow, lessens inflammation.
- Best when used on "hot" or type-A personalities (Chinese medicine), that is: easily overheated and excited, with a red tongue and fast pulse.

FOLKLORE: In the eighteenth century Skullcap was claimed to be a cure for rabies, hence the names "Mad dog" and "Madweed," but that claim was ultimately discredited (although it does relieve some of the symptoms).

INFUSION: Mix 1–2 tsp. dried herb (or 2–3 tsp. fresh) in 1 cup boiling water; infuse 15 minutes. Drink 3 times a day.

TINCTURE: Take 1–2 ml. 2–3 times a day.

IMPORTANT: Do not take during pregnancy, as it may cause miscarriage. Do not exceed recommended doses, as it may cause confusion, stupor, irregular heartbeat, and/or twitching.

SOAPWORT

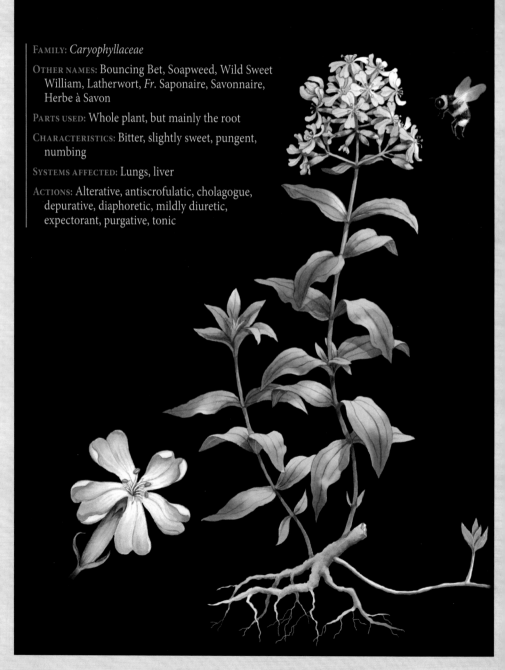

Saponaria officinalis

FAMILY: *Caryophyllaceae*

OTHER NAMES: Bouncing Bet, Soapweed, Wild Sweet William, Latherwort, *Fr.* Saponaire, Savonnaire, Herbe à Savon

PARTS USED: Whole plant, but mainly the root

CHARACTERISTICS: Bitter, slightly sweet, pungent, numbing

SYSTEMS AFFECTED: Lungs, liver

ACTIONS: Alterative, antiscrofulatic, cholagogue, depurative, diaphoretic, mildly diuretic, expectorant, purgative, tonic

A perennial plant often found along roadsides throughout the Maritimes, Soapwort began in this country as a garden plant brought over from Europe and quickly became naturalized. As the name suggests, it has been used since ancient Greek times as a natural cleanser, and is still used today for cleaning delicate fabrics and tapestries, making a soap-like lather when the bruised leaves are agitated in water. It can grow up to 70 cm. high, with round, slightly reddish stems, sparingly branched, and with opposite ovate or lance-shaped leaves that are 3-veined and smooth along the margins. The mildly fragrant pink or whitish flowers which bloom throughout the summer are composed of 5 petals, forming a deep tubular cup, and are frequently double. The fruit is an oblong capsule with 4–5 teeth containing numerous black seeds, which disperse readily. It also has a creeping rootstock, which will quickly take over a garden. Harvest 2- or 3-year-old rhizomes in the spring and dry for later use.

MEDICINAL USES:

Skin itchiness, coughs

- Contains saponins, which can be an irritant to the digestive tract if taken in large doses or over long periods of time. However, taken in small doses for a few days, it can be an effective cough remedy, particularly for dry coughs in bronchitis or pneumonia, as its irritant action causes the body to produce more mucus in the respiratory tract.
- Tonic, induces sweating, increases bile flow, and cleanses the bowel.
- A decoction of the root applied externally can soothe itching skin, and is effective for eczema and psoriasis. Alternatively, the leaves and flowers may be added to the bathwater.
- Once used for rheumatism and joint pain, but is rarely administered internally now.
- Soap may be obtained by boiling the whole plant, especially the root, in water. Best for washing delicate fabrics.

DECOCTION: Soak 4 tbsp. dried root (or 2 tbsp. finely cut fresh) in about 4 cups cold water for 5 hours. Bring to a boil and simmer for 10 minutes. Drink 1 cup 3–4 times a day.

LOTION: For psoriasis and acne, boil 4 cups of water, add 2 cups chopped leaves and root, boil for 15 minutes. Strain and cool before applying.

IMPORTANT: Do not use over long periods of time, as it can cause irritation in the digestive tract. Contains saponins, so use in doses not exceeding 1.5 g of dried rootstock and for a duration of less than 2 weeks.

SOLOMON'S SEAL

Polygonatum pubescens

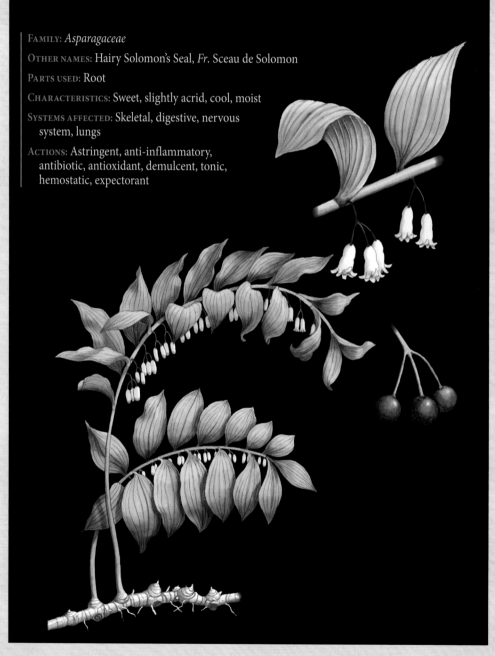

FAMILY: *Asparagaceae*

OTHER NAMES: Hairy Solomon's Seal, *Fr.* Sceau de Solomon

PARTS USED: Root

CHARACTERISTICS: Sweet, slightly acrid, cool, moist

SYSTEMS AFFECTED: Skeletal, digestive, nervous system, lungs

ACTIONS: Astringent, anti-inflammatory, antibiotic, antioxidant, demulcent, tonic, hemostatic, expectorant

The use of Solomon's Seal as a wound-healer dates back several thousand years, and is still popular among herbalists. It is a native perennial herb found in woodlands and often grown in shade gardens throughout eastern Canada. Its graceful, arching stems are between 30–90 cm. tall with elliptical leaves. The leaves are slightly hairy on the underside along the veins, and are arranged alternately along the stem. Its white-to-greenish, dangling, bell-shaped flowers hang from the leaf axis in groups of 1 to 3. The berries are dark blue and considered poisonous. The roots are fleshy with knobby circular scars from the previous year's growth. When harvesting the root in the fall, to avoid killing the plant, dig down gently with your fingers or a trowel until you find the rear portion, which will be away from the next year's bud. Run your fingers under it and cut a few cm. away from the stem, leaving the plant intact. This plant is endangered so it is important to collect it in a sustainable manner.

MEDICINAL USES:

Pulled ligaments and tendons, wounds, bleeding, sore joints, broken bones

- One of nature's best anti-inflammatory herbs for repairing cartilage, tendons, ligaments, sprains, and broken bones, and for chronic problems like arthritis and tendonitis. It tightens or loosens joints as needed, moistening and promoting the production of joint fluid. May also be used as an external remedy for sprains and joint pain when used in an oil infusion.
- Since it is excellent for moistening and lubricating, it can be used in a decoction to loosen mucus when there is a dry cough, bronchitis, or other dry lung condition.
- Helps reduce inflammation in the intestines; soothes irritation.
- Heals wounds and stops bleeding and bruising.
- Great for treating pain, inflammation, and stress, so it works well to treat the symptoms of PMS; mild sedative.
- Lowers blood pressure; antioxidant, lowers cholesterol.
- Soothes an upset stomach.
- Boosts the immune system, increases vitality.

TINCTURE FOR JOINT INJURIES: 7 parts Solomon's Seal, 5 parts each Mullein and Horsetail, and 1 part Goldenseal tinctures.

INFUSION: Steep ½ tsp. of herb in 1 cup hot water for 5 minutes. Take 2–3 times a day. Do not take for more than 7–10 days consecutively, and stop for 3 or 4 days before repeating treatment (if further treatment is necessary).

TINCTURE: Should be extracted in high-proof alcohol to make a tincture. Start with 5 drops a day; increase to up to 12 if necessary for relief.

IMPORTANT: Do not consume berries; they are toxic. Avoid if pregnant or breastfeeding. Do not consume if taking heart medications. Avoid if you are diabetic, as it may decrease blood sugar levels. Do not exceed recommended dose.

ST. JOHN'S WORT

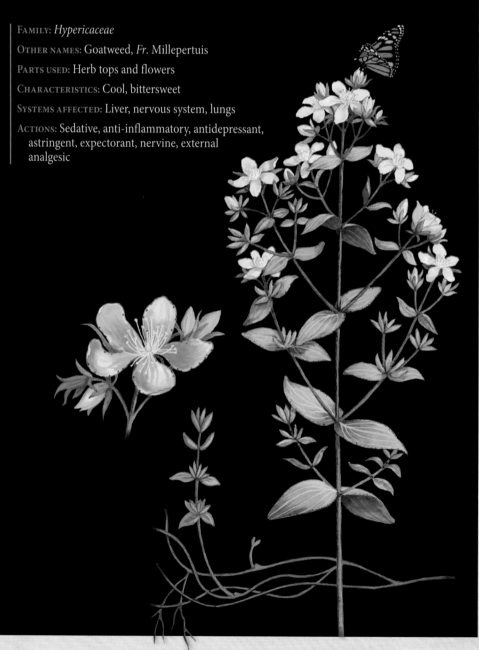

Hypericum perforatum

FAMILY: *Hypericaceae*

OTHER NAMES: Goatweed, *Fr.* Millepertuis

PARTS USED: Herb tops and flowers

CHARACTERISTICS: Cool, bittersweet

SYSTEMS AFFECTED: Liver, nervous system, lungs

ACTIONS: Sedative, anti-inflammatory, antidepressant, astringent, expectorant, nervine, external analgesic

St. John's Wort has been used as a medicinal herb for over two thousand years, with many stories and myths attached to it. It is an herbaceous perennial, growing up to 1 metre high with a central stem branching out into several at the top. The leaves are opposite and have tiny translucent spots, which are actually oil glands. The star-shaped flowers appear from June to August and are yellow with 5 petals and tiny black dots on the calyx and corolla. The root is a creeping rhizome, and the woody stem has 2 longitudinal ridges. It can be found in dry fields and along roadsides. Harvest leaves and flowers as plants bloom. Dry and store in an airtight jar.

MEDICINAL USES:

Nervous system disorders, depression, anxiety, rheumatic and arthritic pain

- Primarily used today internally to relieve symptoms of anxiety and depression, it also helps treat seasonal affective disorder (SAD), PMS, menopause, and insomnia due to the presence of hyperforin, which calms and strengthens the nervous system. It could take 1–3 months of continuous use before results are seen.
- May be effective in easing nerve pain, lower back pain, rheumatism, arthritis, and chronic inflammation.
- An oil or ointment made from the flowers has been used since the Middle Ages as an astringent to heal wounds, sores, bruises, insect bites, and hemorrhoids, and to help prevent and treat inflammation. Also useful for muscle spasms and backaches.
- Indigenous peoples once used it as a tea to protect against tuberculosis and other respiratory ailments, as well as to treat fever, snakebites, and skin problems.
- Contains hypericin, which has been proven an effective antiviral in the treatment of HIV/AIDS, herpes, and hepatitis.
- A cup of infusion before bed can help some children with bedwetting.

FOLKLORE: Named after St. John the Baptist, as it usually flowers around June 24, St. John's Day. Since Ancient Greece its fragrance was believed to chase away evil spirits, and was used for centuries as a charm against witchcraft and in exorcisms. In medieval times, women would pick the herb on St. John's Eve with the dew still on the leaves, as it was believed this would help them find a husband.

INFUSION: Infuse 1 heaping tsp of dried herb in 1 cup of boiling water 10–15 minutes; drink up to 3 times a day.

TINCTURE: Take 1–2 ml. 3 times a day.

OIL: Place flowers in a glass jar and add just enough olive oil to cover. Place jar in a sunny window 2–3 weeks; shake daily. Filter and place in a dark glass container.

IMPORTANT: Excessive use may cause photosensitivity or allergies in some people and animals. Do not take in combination with other drugs, narcotics, alcohol, cold or hay fever medications, birth control, tryptophan, or tyrosine. Do not use during pregnancy.

STINGING NETTLE

Urtica dioica

FAMILY: *Urticaceae*

OTHER NAMES: Common Nettle, *Fr.* Grande Ortie

PARTS USED: Leaves, root

CHARACTERISTICS: Bland, slightly bitter, warm, drying

SYSTEMS AFFECTED: Lungs, liver, urinary tract

ACTIONS: Diuretic, astringent, tonic, hemostatic, galactagogue, expectorant, nutritive, antiseptic, anti-inflammatory

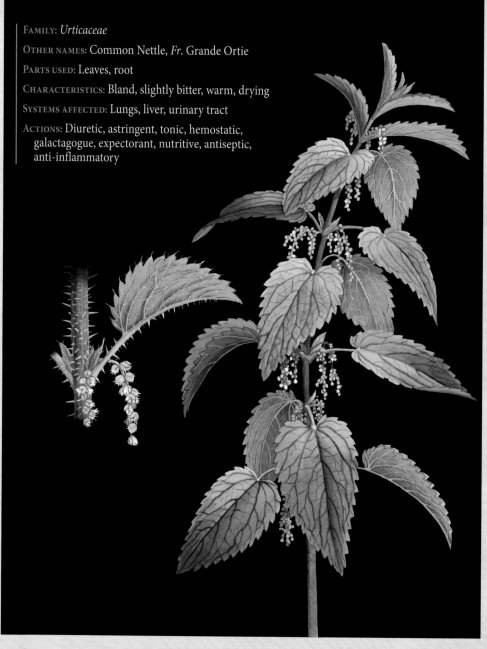

Although this plant has a bad reputation for its stinging hairs, it is one of the best medicinal herbs if properly handled, and has a wide variety of applications. A perennial that grows 30–90 cm. high, it has oval leaves, which are opposite, tapered to a point, and finely toothed. The roots are creeping rhizomes so it multiplies easily; the flowers are greenish and hang in branched clusters. The stiff hairs covering the entire plant contain a small amount of formic acid, which is what causes the sting, but rubbing Dock leaf or Plantain onto affected areas can neutralize it. The plant loses its sting after it's been dried or cooked, or even if stored in the refrigerator for a day or so. It is usually found in waste places and ditches where the soil is moist; gather with rubber gloves in the spring or early summer when the leaves are free of dew; hang to dry in a shaded area for later use.

MEDICINAL USES:

Arthritis, asthma, bronchitis, eczema, cystitis, stagnant mucus, enlarged prostate, stones, diarrhea, hemorrhoids

- Makes a wonderful spring tonic, cleansing herb, and blood purifier. It is high in vitamins C and A, potassium, and iron. The young leaves steamed taste a bit like spinach, and when eaten over a long period can benefit those with anemia or depleted energy from loss of fluids. Also, when steamed for 30 minutes, juice may be squeezed out and 1 tbsp. taken every hour to reduce heavy menstruation and stop internal bleeding.
- After childbirth, Stinging Nettle tea may be used to promote milk production and build up the blood in cases of anemia and depleted energy from loss of fluids. Combines well with Raspberry leaf.
- Contains a high amount of sterols, especially in the root, and may be effective in treating enlarged prostate and stimulating the white blood cells to counteract inflammation.
- Removes stagnant mucus in the lungs and sinuses, so it is useful for treating asthma, pneumonia, pleurisy, bronchitis, and allergies. Traditionally, it was burned and the smoke inhaled to treat lung infections.
- Useful for lowering uric acid levels, it can prevent or treat gout and kidney or bladder stones. Good for urinary tract infections.
- Relieves diarrhea, dysentery, hemorrhoids, and mucus in the stool, and cold, damp conditions.
- Compresses reduce pain of arthritis, rheumatism. Purposely stinging oneself causes increased blood flow to the skin, relieving inflammation of the joints.

OTHER USES: Stem fibres were once used to weave fabric, clothing, rope, and netting.

INFUSION: Mix 1–2 tsp. dried herb in 1 cup boiling water; infuse 10–15 min. Drink 3 times a day.

TINCTURE: Take 6–12 drops 3 times a day.

IMPORTANT: Handle with gloves. Not recommended for pregnant women. Could interfere with blood-thinning drugs or diuretic drugs. May lower blood pressure.

SUNDEW (Round-leafed)

Drosera rotundifolia

FAMILY: *Droseraceae*

OTHER NAMES: Dew plant, Red root, Herba rosellae, *Fr.* Rosée du soleil

PARTS USED: Aerial

CHARACTERISTICS: Bitter, acrid

SYSTEMS AFFECTED: Lungs, stomach

ACTIONS: Antispasmodic, antibiotic, demulcent, expectorant

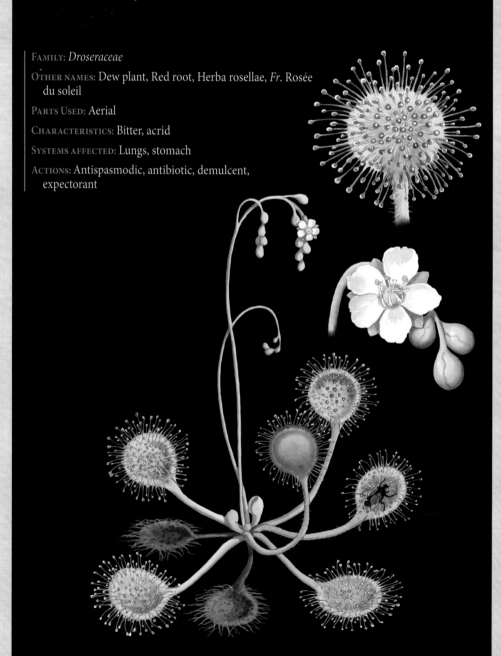

This tiny native aquatic plant can be found in acidic peaty soil alongside ponds, and rivers, or in damp woods. An insectivore (or insect-eating) perennial, its leaves grow close to the ground in basal rosettes and are covered with red glandular hairs, which exude sticky mucilaginous drops that resemble morning dew. They lure and catch insects, holding on to them as their leaves fold over and digest them. The tiny 5-petalled white or pink flowers emerge from the middle of the rosette on erect leafless stems 5–15 cm. high, and appear in summer or early fall. This plant is endangered, so it should be left where it is unless it's cultivated or growing in abundance in the area. Gather in midsummer and air-dry for later use.

MEDICINAL USES:

Tuberculosis, coughs, asthma, whooping cough, bronchitis, warts, stomach ulcers

- Its antispasmodic and antibiotic properties make it effective in treating lung infections with dry coughs and inflamed respiratory tract issues. It has a relaxing effect on the involuntary muscles and thins the mucus, making it easier to cough up, reducing coughing spasms, and soothing tissues.
- The juice of the plant contains enzymes that will dissolve warts, bunions, and corns.
- Has been reported to have aphrodisiac effects.

FOLKLORE AND OTHER USES: Was once employed in Sweden to sour milk in the making of cheese. The "dew" on the leaves was once believed to endow long life or restore youth to anyone who drank it.

INFUSION: Add 1 tsp. dried herb to 1 cup steaming water; infuse 10–15 minutes. Strain and drink 3 times a day.

TINCTURE: Take 5–15 drops, 3 times a day.

IMPORTANT: Do not exceed recommended doses. Do not take if pregnant or breastfeeding.

TANSY

Tanacetum vulgare

FAMILY: *Asteraceae*

OTHER NAMES: Golden buttons, Stinking Willie, *Fr.* Tanaisie commune

PARTS USED: Aerial

CHARACTERISTICS: Bitter

SYSTEMS AFFECTED: Circulatory, digestive, reproductive

ACTIONS: Anthelmintic, antispasmodic, antiseptic, anti-inflammatory, emmenagogue, insecticide, carminative, vermifuge

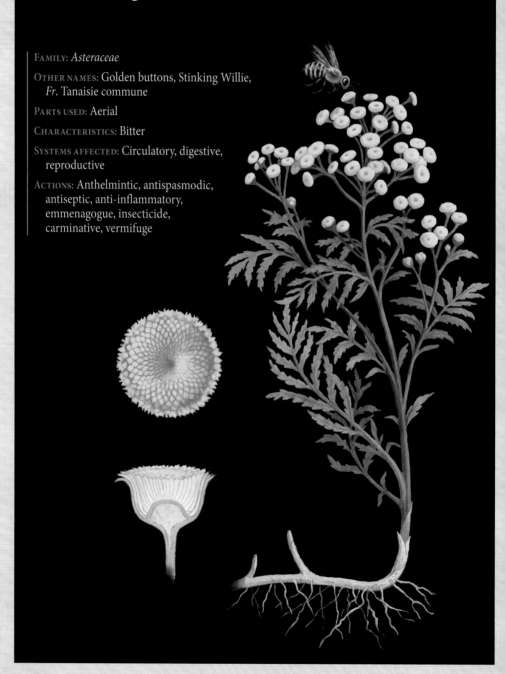

Tansy is an aromatic perennial that is rarely used any more as a medicinal herb due to its thujone content, which can be toxic in large doses—although in small amounts it can be quite effective to remove parasites. It has a hardy, erect stem about 75 cm. high, which is grooved and angular, with fern-like, feathery, alternate leaves. It is distinguished by its round, yellow, composite flowers that grow in clusters and look like small buttons, with an odour much like a mixture of Camphor and Rosemary. It blooms from July to September, and is found in fields and along roadsides. Harvest as it is coming into flower and dry for later use.

MEDICINAL USES:

Expels worms, brings on menstruation

- Fresh leaves crushed and applied to skin can relieve swelling, bruises, varicose veins, scabies, and lice.
- When heated in a fomentation, it will relieve rheumatism, gout, neuralgia, and muscle pain.
- A weak infusion stimulates digestion, aids in dyspepsia, and relieves flatulence.
- Promotes menstruation. Not for use during pregnancy.
- Seeds and aerial parts once used in infusions to expel worms, particularly in children.
- Strengthens the heart and reduces blood pressure.

OTHER USES: As a strewing herb it was scattered on floors as a disinfectant and to repel insects. Used as a companion herb in gardens to repel many destructive insects. When dried, the flowers last a long time in bouquets. Flowers were once used as a dye.

FOLKLORE: Leaves once used in Tansy cakes throughout England during Easter; its bitter taste helped cleanse the body after Lent and symbolized the suffering of the Jews at Passover. Irish folklore claimed bathing in Tansy and salt would cure joint pain.

INFUSION: Mix ½–1 tsp. dried herb and 1 cup of boiling water. Infuse 10–15 minutes; drink no more than 2 times daily.

IMPORTANT: Can be toxic in large quantities. Do not use over long periods of time or in large doses. Use only under supervision of a certified herbalist. Do not take during pregnancy, as it can cause miscarriage.

TURTLEHEAD (White)

Chelone glabra

FAMILY: *Plantaginaceae*

OTHER NAMES: Balmony, Snakehead, *Fr*: Galane glabre, Tête de tortue

PARTS USED: Aerial

CHARACTERISTICS: Bitter, pungent

SYSTEMS AFFECTED: Digestive

ACTIONS: Anthelmintic, antibilious, anti-inflammatory, antiemetic, aperient, cholagogue, tonic

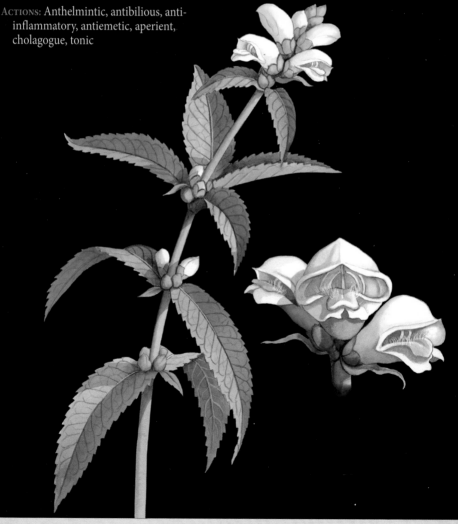

Turtlehead or Balmony is a native perennial that has been used in North American folk medicine for centuries. Its name comes from Greek mythology, which tells of a nymph named Chelone who insulted the gods and was subsequently turned into a turtle. The plant is found in wetlands, ditches, and woodlands across eastern Canada, and can grow up to 1 metre tall. Its erect stems end in clusters of white or pinkish, tubular, 2-lipped flowers shaped like a turtle's head. The lance-shaped leaves are notched, and grow opposite to each other along the smooth, square stem. Gather when in full bloom, from August to October, and dry for later use.

MEDICINAL USES:

Sluggish liver, gallstones, nausea, hemorrhoids, anorexia

- Very bitter herb that acts as a tonic for the liver and digestive system by increasing digestive fluids to stimulate the appetite and aid in the treatment of liver disease, gallbladder problems and stones. Also relieves nausea and vomiting, cramps, worms, and constipation. Tonifies the digestive tract and helps in the treatment of anorexia nervosa.
- Used in ointments to treat hemorrhoids, herpes, inflamed breasts, eczema, sores, and wounds. Relieves itching and inflammation.
- Remedy has been used by Indigenous peoples as a liver tonic, to expel worms, to treat jaundice, malaria, and fever, and in various salves for skin problems.

INFUSION: 2 tsp. dried herb in 1 cup of boiling water; steep 10–15 minutes. Drink 1–3 times a day.

OIL INFUSION: Use fresh leaves, pack into a Mason jar up to two-thirds full. Fill with olive oil and let sit about 6 weeks, shaking often. Use in salves.

IMPORTANT: Avoid during pregnancy. May decrease sexual drive in men.

VALERIAN

Valeriana officinalis

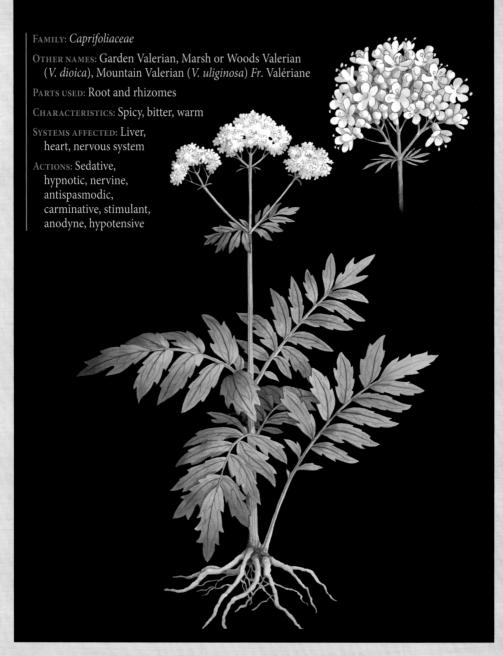

FAMILY: *Caprifoliaceae*

OTHER NAMES: Garden Valerian, Marsh or Woods Valerian (*V. dioica*), Mountain Valerian (*V. uliginosa*) *Fr.* Valériane

PARTS USED: Root and rhizomes

CHARACTERISTICS: Spicy, bitter, warm

SYSTEMS AFFECTED: Liver, heart, nervous system

ACTIONS: Sedative, hypnotic, nervine, antispasmodic, carminative, stimulant, anodyne, hypotensive

Valerian's genus is comprised of about 150 species, the most widely used in herbology being the Garden Valerian (*V. officinalis*), which is native to Europe and Asia. It is now cultivated in eastern Canada but has also escaped to the wild, and is the species typically used in formulas for insomnia. Attaining a height of 1.2–1.5 metres, this perennial often takes several years to produce flowers, which can be pink or white and fragrant, growing atop a grooved, hollow, slightly hairy stem in two or more pairs of clusters or cymes. The leaves are in pairs of lance-shaped toothed segments growing somewhat opposite with a slightly hairy underside. The plant sends out runners that spread quickly, and the roots give off a fetid odour, somewhat like smelly socks. The root is more potent if kept from flowering and should be at least 2 years old; dig it up after the leaves have died down in the fall. Tincture and infusions are best made from the fresh root, but the roots may also be dried for later use.

MEDICINAL USES:

Insomnia, hypertension, menstrual cramps, eczema

- Eases pain and promotes sleep; helps with restless leg syndrome, anxiety, tension, and strained nerves. Should be used over a period of several weeks to be most effective.
- Some studies show it may have a calming effect on people with obsessive-compulsive disorder (OCD) and children with hyperactivity. Often combined with Lemon Balm.
- Relieves menstrual cramps, intestinal colic, muscle spasms or cramps.
- Reduces blood pressure and has a calming effect on agitated people. May be effective in the treatment of epilepsy.
- Externally, an infusion can be used as a wash or compress to treat eczema and minor injuries, or to relieve muscle spasms.

OTHER USES: May be used to speed up bacterial activity in compost heaps as well as being a good fertilizer in gardens, attracting earthworms and adding phosphorus to the soil. Cats and rats are often attracted to it.

TINCTURE: Take 1–5 ml. an hour or two before bedtime (start with a smaller dose in case it causes headache).

IMPORTANT: No known side effects, although it's not advisable to exceed usage for longer than 3 months. Do not take with other sedatives.

VERVAIN (Blue)

Verbena hastata

FAMILY: *Verbenaceae*

OTHER NAMES: Blue verbena, Indian Hyssop, Swamp verbena, Herba sacra *Fr*. Verveine bleue

PARTS USED: Aerial

CHARACTERISTICS: Cold, bitter, drying

SYSTEMS AFFECTED: Liver/gallbladder, spleen, nervous system, cardiovascular, urinary

ACTIONS: Nervine, diuretic, expectorant, emmenagogue, tonic, emetic (in large doses), astringent, diaphoretic, antispasmodic, febrifuge, galactagogue, anticatarrhal, vulnerary, tranquilizer

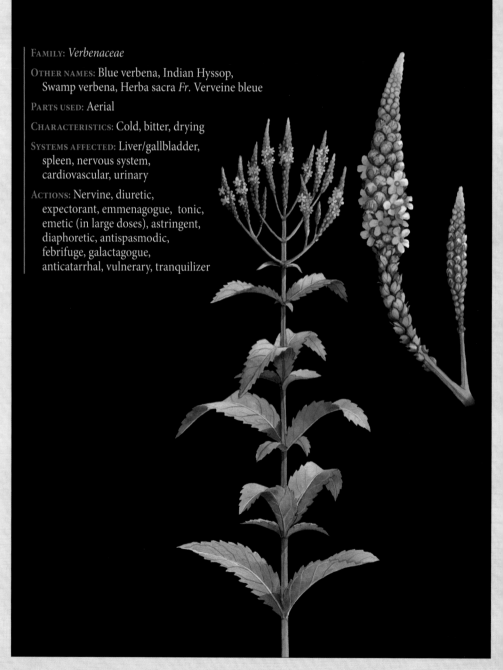

This common weed native to North America is similar in medicinal properties to the European variety *Verbena officinalis*. It is a tall, erect, branching perennial that grows from 0.6–1.5 metres high with intense blue–violet flower spikes. It has a reddish, square stem and opposite lanceolate leaves that are conspicuously veined and coarsely serrated. It blooms from mid- to late summer, each flower spike being up to 12.5 cm. long, the individual flowers having 5 lobes and no noticeable scent. It grows in ditches, along roadsides, and in pastures throughout the Maritimes but also is often grown in gardens to attract butterflies. Harvest when the plants come into bloom, tincture fresh or dry quickly in a cool dark place for later use in teas.

MEDICINAL USES:

Colds, headaches, pain, anxiety, bleeding gums, arthritis

- Clears up chest congestion, colds, fevers, chronic bronchitis, sore throat, and other respiratory infections.
- Muscle relaxant and pain reliever; anti-inflammatory, it helps to relieve stress headaches and swelling and inflammation from gout or arthritis.
- Eliminates toxins and helps protect the liver and kidneys, relieving pain from kidney stones and bladder infections.
- Used as a relaxing nervine, to reduce stress and anxiety and help with insomnia, as well as for tension in the stomach due to suppression of emotions.
- Gentle astringent for soothing inflamed and bleeding gums. Helps teething babies.
- Promotes milk production in nursing mothers, balances women's hormones; good for menstrual pain, PMS, and hot flashes.
- Generally a good herb for "Type A" uptight workaholic personalities, who have trouble sitting still.

FOLKLORE: Once believed to have magical properties, druids and sorcerers used the European variety in their rites and incantations; it was used in love charms as it was said to have aphrodisiac qualities. Called *Herba sacra*, priests used it in rituals, as it was supposedly used to staunch the wounds of Jesus. It was often worn around the neck for good luck and to ward off headaches.

INFUSION: Because of its bitter taste, it's best blended with other herbs like Chamomile, or for headaches with Goldenrod flowers and Mullein. For nerves, mix 4 parts Skullcap, 2 parts Motherwort, and 1 part Blue Vervain.

IMPORTANT: Slight nausea and danger of miscarriage if taken in extremely large doses.

VIOLET (Sweet)

Viola odorata

FAMILY: *Violaceae* (Violet)

OTHER NAMES: Blue violet, *Fr.* Violette

PARTS USED: Aerial

CHARACTERISTICS: Sweet, mild but pleasantly bitter, cool

SYSTEMS AFFECTED: Lungs, stomach, liver, heart

PROPERTIES: Demulcent, expectorant, astringent, alterative, febrifuge, antiseptic, vulnerary, antispasmodic, anodyne, anti-scrofulous

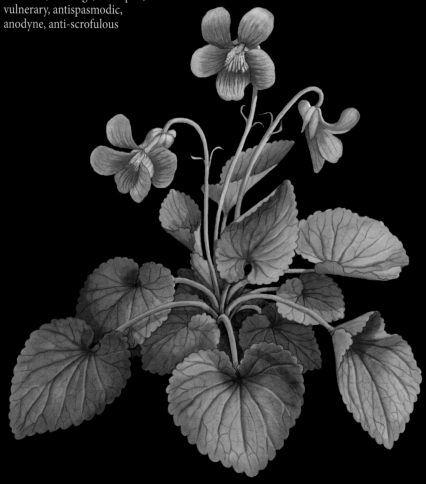

Violets are pretty little creeping perennials, some of which are native to Europe and others to North America, and belong to a genus of over 900 species, all with similar medicinal uses. Many foreign species have now naturalized throughout most of North America and they are one of the first flowers to appear in the spring, traditionally symbolizing rebirth and bringing joy at the end of a long winter. Its leaves are heart-shaped, dark green, with scalloped edges and grow in rosettes close to the ground. The fragrant flowers can be anywhere from deep purple to blue, pinkish, or even white. They are 5-petalled with a yellow beard in the centre and bloom from April to June. Oddly enough, Violet produces a second kind of flower later in the summer, growing colourless and hidden underground. Although these flowers never see the light of day, they do produce viable seeds. If you pick only the leaves and flowers without disturbing the underground parts, Violets will continue to produce leaves all summer. Eat only the aerial parts, use fresh or dry for later use, storing in a glass jar away from heat and light.

MEDICINAL USES:

Dryness, inflammation, constipation, swollen glands, mastitis

- Very nourishing, rich in vitamins A and C, and minerals, and may be added to Nettles for people with a dry constitution. Contains mucilage, which coats tissues and eases inflammation. Will soothe a sore throat or loosen mucous from the lungs when a cough is dry and unproductive.
- Laxative, the plant lubricates the intestines in cases of constipation.
- May be used in eyewash to lubricate dry eyes.
- Chewed leaves can be applied to corns to soften skin or used as a poultice for hot, inflamed skin eruptions, or bug bites.
- May be used in oil for swollen glands or mastitis, massaged into the area. This is best complemented with an infusion taken internally. Acts as a lymphatic stimulant.
- Topically, it is anti-inflammatory and can be used as a compress, infused oil, or salve to soothe dry or irritated skin, abrasions, insect bites, eczema, and hemorrhoids.
- Has a relaxing effect on the nervous system; contains methyl salicylate, a pain reliever, although in small quantity.

INFUSION: Mix 1 tbsp. dried (or 2 tbsp. minced fresh herb) steeped in 2 cups freshly boiled water for 10 minutes, or overnight. Strain and enjoy. May be combined with equal parts Dandelion leaf, Nettle, Red Clover, and Mint for a highly nutritious tea.

IMPORTANT: Roots should not be eaten as they can cause nausea and vomiting.

WATERPEPPER

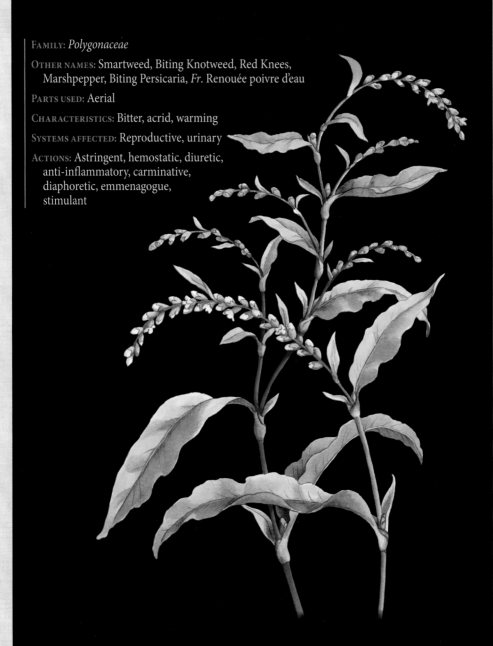

Persicaria (Polygonum) hydropiper

FAMILY: *Polygonaceae*

OTHER NAMES: Smartweed, Biting Knotweed, Red Knees, Marshpepper, Biting Persicaria, *Fr.* Renouée poivre d'eau

PARTS USED: Aerial

CHARACTERISTICS: Bitter, acrid, warming

SYSTEMS AFFECTED: Reproductive, urinary

ACTIONS: Astringent, hemostatic, diuretic, anti-inflammatory, carminative, diaphoretic, emmenagogue, stimulant

W aterpepper or Smartweed is just one of a large family of similar weeds growing throughout North America. It is an annual native to Europe that grows in damp muddy areas, ditches, and along riverbanks, and has a bitter peppery taste. It can reach 30–50 cm. in height with branched stems and dark green, lance-shaped leaves with undulate edges and glands on the underside. The tiny pink or greenish flowers are arranged on terminal spikes, and the fruit is triangular, flat, and dark brown. It is harvested in summer during flowering and dried in the shade, but is more potent if used fresh.

MEDICINAL USES:

Diarrhea, heavy menstrual bleeding, stomach upset, hemorrhoids

- Astringent properties make it useful for treating diarrhea; reduces gas and eases colic.
- Leaves contain rutin, which helps strengthen capillaries and prevents bleeding. Good for hemorrhoids.
- Regulates excessive menstrual bleeding and menstrual irregularities.
- Poultice treats swollen, inflamed areas, minor cuts and bleeding, and slow-healing wounds.
- Used in formulas for treating respiratory ailments.

OTHER USES: As a flavouring for soups or salads, it adds a strong peppery taste. It loses most of its flavour when cooked, so add just before serving.

IMPORTANT: Do not use if pregnant—may cause miscarriage. Use only in moderate doses. Ingestion of large amounts may cause irritation of the digestive system. Plant sap may also cause skin irritation in some people.

WILD LETTUCE

Lactuca serriola

FAMILY: *Asteraceae*

OTHER NAMES: Prickly Lettuce, Compass Plant, China Lettuce, *Fr.* Laitue scariole

PARTS USED: Leaves, dried sap

CHARACTERISTICS: Bitter, cold

SYSTEMS AFFECTED: Nervous, reproductive, lungs

ACTIONS: Narcotic, sedative, antispasmodic, expectorant, nervine, diuretic, diaphoretic

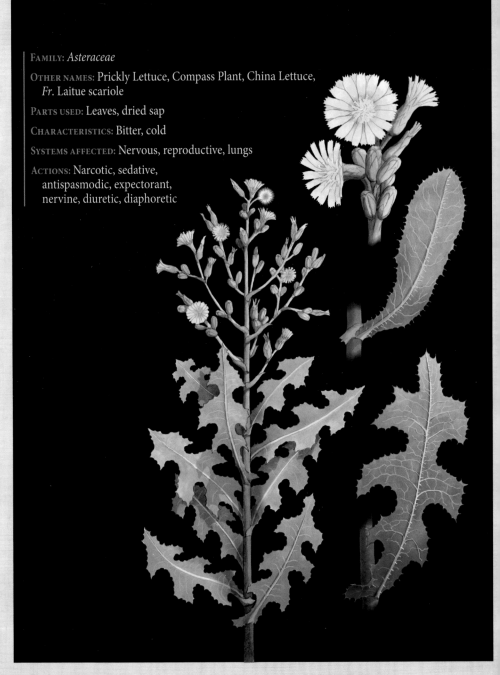

Wild or Prickly Lettuce is an annual or biennial herb, originally from Europe, which is related to many different species scattered throughout North America, all having the same or similar properties. It has a smooth stem growing upright from a large white taproot, 30.5 cm. to 2 metres high. Its leaves are prickly along the edges and on the underside mid-vein, and are either lobed or oblong. Both leaves and stems contain a milky latex sap (although less than its European cousin *L. virosa*), which oozes out when cut and when dried is often used as a mild narcotic. Basal leaves often twist to face the sun, pointing north and south. The light-yellow composite flowers are similar to a small dandelion and bloom from July to September. It is easily mistaken for Sow Thistle, which has no prickles on the underside vein, but it is also edible. Wild Lettuce can be found along roadsides and in waste places, and should be gathered in spring or early summer, before flowering, for teas or salads; wait until flowering to collect the sap. Should be tinctured fresh.

MEDICINAL USES:

Insomnia, anxiety, coughs, colic

- Sap contains lactucarium, which is a mild sedative. Sometimes called Wild Opium, Wild Lettuce was once used as a substitute for opium, although the effects are a lot milder. It can relieve anxiety, reduce pain, and promote sleep. Traditionally, the leaves were dried and smoked as tobacco, or the sap collected and dried for later use.
- Antispasmodic and expectorant, it relieves spasms, colic and chronic coughs, asthma, and bronchitis.
- Promotes sweating and urine production.
- Some believe it reduces the pain and severity of migraine headaches.
- Relieves menstrual pain and may help women who have trouble conceiving.
- Young leaves may be eaten raw or lightly steamed.
- Sap may be applied externally to get rid of warts.

FOLKLORE: Pagans use Wild Lettuce as incense for divination.

INFUSION: 1–2 tsp. leaves in 1 cup boiling water; infuse 10–15 minutes.

TINCTURE: Up to 30 drops per day, taken before bed.

IMPORTANT: Do not use in large doses; may cause stomach upset. Will relax muscles and cause drowsiness and sleep, so consume only before bedtime.

WILD ROSE

Rosa blanda (Meadow rose)
Rosa canina (Dog rose, Briar rose)
Rosa carolina (Carolina rose)
Rosa nitida (New England rose)
Rosa palustris (Swamp rose)
Rosa rugosa (Japanese rose)
Rosa virginiana (Virginia rose)

FAMILY: *Rosaceae*

PARTS USED: Roots, flowers, fruit (hips), bark

CHARACTERISTICS: Sweet, astringent

ACTIONS: Antiseptic, anti-inflammatory, antispasmodic, antioxidant, antiparasitic, sedative, emmenagogue, diuretic, laxative

Wild Rose, known as the "Queen of Flowers," has been cultivated for thousands of years, not just for its beautiful flowers but also for use in perfumes, cosmetics, and medicines. There are hundreds of varieties growing in North America. The most commonly used for medicinal purposes is the Dog Rose (*R. canina*), which was introduced from Eurasia, but any of our native species have similar properties. An upright perennial shrub, it can grow anywhere from 1.2–2.7 metres tall. The fragrant flowers are 4–6 cm. in diameter, have 5 petals, and vary in colour from white or light pink to a deep fuchsia. The leaves are pinnate and notched, with 5 to 7 leaves, and the stems covered in sharp thorns. The fruit, or "hips," which appear in the fall, resemble small tomatoes, those of the Dog Rose being slightly more elongated than other varieties. They should be picked in the fall when bright red, and the seeds and tiny hairs inside should be removed before consuming, as they are irritant. The roots should be dug up in the spring. Petals are most potent when in bud; remove the calyx and stamens and dry gently until crisp for later use. (If not dried long enough they will grow mouldy after a few weeks.)

MEDICINAL USES:

Wounds, menstrual problems, eye irritations, urinary tract infections, sadness, colds, fevers

- Hips: High in vitamin C, as well as A, B3, D, and E, they are rich in antioxidants and work to reduce inflammation. They can be used in cold remedies, or to reduce pain from arthritis, gout, or sore muscles.
- Petals: Mildly sedative, gladden the heart; antiseptic treatment for wounds, bruising, or rashes; taken internally as an infusion for sore throat, ulcers, stomach upset; can help lower fevers and also help ease heavy periods, infertility, and irregular menstruation.
- Roots: Most often used in Indigenous remedies, the steeped roots or hips are used to treat eye inflammation. Root decoctions ease cramping and heavy menstruation; may be used as an aphrodisiac.
- Bark: Used in a decoction to ease upset stomach and diarrhea.

OTHER USES: Petals may be sprinkled on salads, or added to potpourri.

INFUSION: Add 2–4 tsp. dried petals to 1 cup of boiling water. Steep 10–15 minutes. Add honey for coughs.

ROSE HIP TEA: Simmer 4 tsp. Rose hips in 1 cup water for 5 minutes. Add Mint leaves or Ginger root if desired.

HONEY: Add several unopened leaf and flower buds to a jar of honey; let sit for at least 1 week before using. This may be added to teas with lemon for a good cold remedy, or simply eaten from a spoon as a sore throat remedy or aphrodisiac.

ROSE WATER: Pick the petals on a sunny day, put into a pan and immerse in spring water. Cover and put on low heat until it simmers, then turn down lower and leave 10 minutes. Turn off heat and let sit overnight. Strain and add ¼ of the volume of vodka. Bottle and store in a cool, dark place. Use as a skin toner or flavouring in cooking.

IMPORTANT: Remove hairs from inside the fruit/hips, as they can cause irritation of the throat and digestive tract.

WILD THYME

Thymus serpyllum
Thymus pulegioides

FAMILY: *Lamiaceae*

OTHER NAMES: Creeping thyme, Garden thyme, *Fr.* Thym

PARTS USED: Aerial

CHARACTERISTICS: Spicy, warm, slightly bitter, drying

SYSTEMS AFFECTED: Liver, lungs, stomach

ACTIONS: Carminative, antiseptic, expectorant, antitussive, sedative, anthelmintic, antispasmodic, diaphoretic, tonic

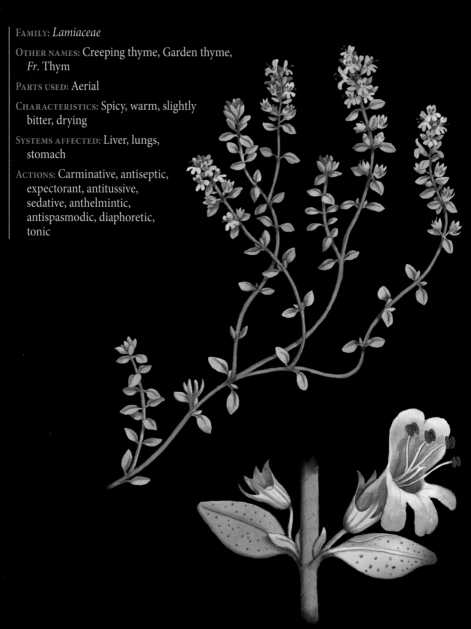

This common garden herb originated in Europe but now also grows wild throughout the Maritimes, with similar properties to the garden variety (*Thymus vulgaris*) although to a lesser degree. It is a perennial evergreen shrub, but rarely grows higher than about 10 cm. in the wild, creeping along roadsides and lawns in dense masses. The stems and roots are woody, reddish brown, with tiny green oval leaves set in opposite pairs. The pink or mauve flowers bloom from early summer to early fall, and the entire plant gives off a distinct fragrance that can be detected from several metres away. It should be gathered when in full flower and can be dried for later use.

MEDICINAL USES:

Gastrointestinal problems, headaches, coughs and colds, mouth and throat infections, menstrual cramps; powerful antiseptic

- The essential oil is a potent antibiotic, anti-fungal, and antiseptic, but use with caution, as it is very strong and should be diluted with almond or other oils. Can be applied to insect bites, scabies, infected wounds, athlete's foot, or the breasts in cases of mastitis. When combined with lavender oil and rubbed on the skin it warms the area, increases circulation, and relieves pain from rheumatism or strained muscles; can be rubbed on the chest for coughs and congestion.
- The plant contains thymol and carvacrol, which help relieve menstrual cramps, relax muscles, and relieve tension headaches.
- Infusions are used to help stomach and bowel disorders such as indigestion, gas, diarrhea, food poisoning, candida, and sluggish digestion.
- Traditionally used as a medicine for dry, unproductive coughs. Loosens phlegm; helps with stubborn bronchitis. May also be used in a bath to help with a cough or to ease muscle aches.
- Infusion used as a mouthwash to treat gum infections, or as a gargle for sore throat, coughs, and laryngitis.

FOLKLORE: Scottish highlanders made a tea from Wild Thyme to give them strength and courage and to prevent nightmares. Pliny the Elder (23 AD–79 AD), a Roman naturalist and author, claimed it to be a cure for snakebites. In the Middle Ages it was included in a recipe that would enable a person to see fairies.

INFUSION: Mix 3 or 4 tsp. of fresh or dried herb in 4 cups boiling water. Cover and steep 10–15 minutes. For coughs, add a demulcent such as Mullein or Coltsfoot and some honey. Take 1 tbsp. at a time throughout the day.

IMPORTANT: May act as a uterine stimulant. Avoid using if pregnant. The essential oil is very concentrated and irritant; should be diluted before using.

YARROW

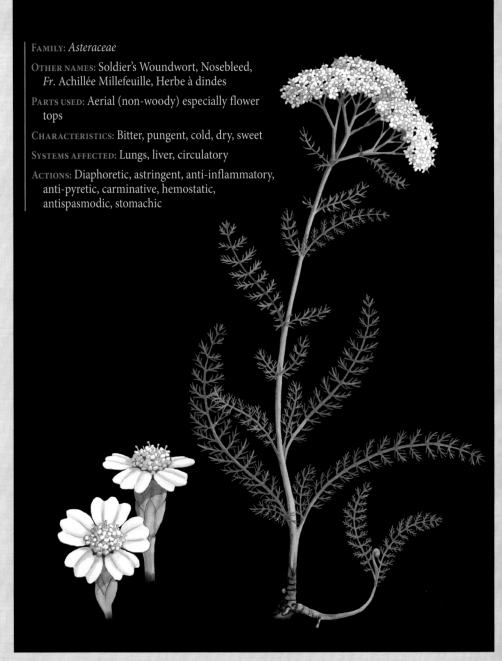

Achillea millefolium

FAMILY: *Asteraceae*

OTHER NAMES: Soldier's Woundwort, Nosebleed,
Fr. Achillée Millefeuille, Herbe à dindes

PARTS USED: Aerial (non-woody) especially flower
tops

CHARACTERISTICS: Bitter, pungent, cold, dry, sweet

SYSTEMS AFFECTED: Lungs, liver, circulatory

ACTIONS: Diaphoretic, astringent, anti-inflammatory,
anti-pyretic, carminative, hemostatic,
antispasmodic, stomachic

This common perennial weed found throughout North America has been popular as a medicinal herb for centuries. It gets its name from the Greek myth of Achilles, who was invulnerable to arrows except on his heel, and it was traditionally used to stop the bleeding of soldier's wounds on battlefields. It grows 20–90 cm. tall, with stems branching near the top and alternate, highly segmented, feathery leaves. At the top of the stalk are clusters of white or pink daisy-like flowers with 5 petals, which bloom throughout the summer and fall. The plant grows in fields and on roadsides but is more potent if found in stony, sandy soils, and should be harvested early in the summer. Avoid using the woody stalks and mature leaves, as there is less medicine in these parts.

MEDICINAL USES

Wounds, fevers, poor digestion, urinary tract infections, menstrual cramps, hemorrhoids

- Has been used as a wound remedy since Roman times, being especially good for deep wounds that bleed profusely. It will stop hemorrhaging, while at the same time breaking up congealed blood or bruises. May be used internally as an infusion or tincture, or externally as a poultice. The Mi'kmaq use it in teas or pound the plant into a pulp to treat sprains, bruises, and wounds. A leaf placed in the nostril can stop a nosebleed.
- Relieves fever by causing sweating, so is therefore good for colds and flu, especially in children. May be used along with Peppermint and Elder flower.
- Used for chronic urinary tract infections, incontinence.
- Bitter, it stimulates stomach acids to aid digestion of fats and proteins, helps with symptoms of heartburn. Soothes mild diarrhea and dysentery.
- Helps ease menstrual cramps and regulates irregular periods.
- Tones the blood vessels; relieves bleeding hemorrhoids and varicose veins, as well as internal bleeding and ulcers. Also tones the mucus membranes of the digestive tract, and is therefore particularly useful for treating dysentery, colitis, and leaky gut.
- May be used in a sitz bath to help with uterine fibroids, varicose veins, hemorrhoids, leukorrhea, rashes, or eczema.
- Anti-inflammatory, it eases pain of osteoarthritis.
- Good for countering the side effects from radiation therapy and hot flashes.

INFUSION: Mix 1–2 tsp. dried herb in 1 cup boiling water; infuse 10–15 minutes. Drink hot 3 times a day. For fevers, drink hourly, and add Elder flower or Spearmint if desired.

TINCTURE: Take 2–4 ml. 3 times a day.

SITZ BATH: Steep ½ cup whole cut herb in cold water overnight. Bring to boil, strain, and then add to bathwater.

IMPORTANT: Avoid using over a long period of time. When symptoms subside, stop using it. Not advised during pregnancy.

YELLOW DOCK

Rumex crispus

FAMILY: *Polygonaceae*

OTHER NAMES: Curly dock, Broad-leafed dock, Sour dock, *Fr.* Oseille crépue, Patience crépue

PARTS USED: Primarily the root, but also the stems, leaves, and seeds

CHARACTERISTICS: Bitter, cold, dry

SYSTEMS AFFECTED: Liver, intestines, lymphatic, kidneys

ACTIONS: Astringent, laxative, alterative, tonic, hepatic, cholagogue

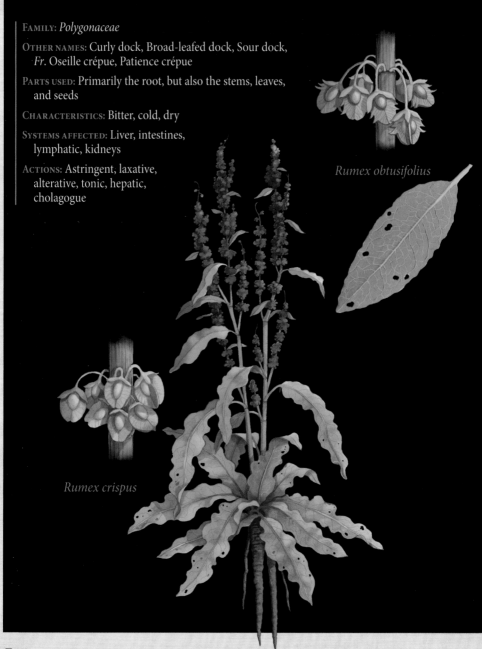

Rumex obtusifolius

Rumex crispus

This common perennial weed is native to Europe and Africa but is now found throughout most of North America. As its various names imply, it has broad, wavy, crinkled leaves, which are crisp around the edges. Its long taproot is usually not forked, and is yellow inside with a thick rusty brown bark. Its close relative, *Rumex obtusifolius*, or Bitter Dock, has similar properties, but is distinguished by its wider, flat leaves and tiny spikes on its seedpods. Both are tenacious weeds often despised by gardeners, as each root must be dug out in its entirety—even the smallest piece left in the ground will produce another plant. The stem grows up to 0.9 metres high, with green flower spikes branching off at intervals, producing an abundance of rust-coloured seed spikes in late summer and fall. The roots should be dug up in late summer or early fall; clean well and split lengthwise before drying.

MEDICINAL USES:
Liver sluggishness, constipation, skin irritations, anemia, throat and gum inflammation, eczema, arthritis

- Digestive tonic that acts specifically on the liver, gallbladder, and kidneys, promoting bile production, cleansing, and assisting in the digestion of fats and proteins. This in turn improves conditions related to a sluggish liver including acne, psoriasis, headaches, constipation, arthritis, and long-term chronic diseases of the intestinal tract. Good for chronic constipation as it gently stimulates peristalsis and increases mucous production in the colon. Add fennel or cumin seed for flavour if desired. Avoid long-term use (preferably no longer than 1 week).
- The plant contains many nutrients, but is particularly rich in iron. Cleanses and nourishes the blood, aids in increasing the absorption of minerals in the intestines, and is helpful in formulas as a remedy for anemia. Strengthens capillaries, helps reduce hemorrhoids and varicose veins, and stems internal bleeding.
- Decoction of the boiled stems or roots can be used in an ointment made with beeswax and olive oil to relieve itching, eczema, psoriasis, or other skin irritations. The decoction also works topically as an antiseptic and astringent to treat wounds, swellings, burns, hemorrhoids, and insect bites. Young shoots, when rubbed on the skin, will help soothe Nettle stings.
- Commonly used for inflammation of the nasal passage, throat, and gums, as well as to treat coughs and bronchitis.

DECOCTION: Mix 1 tsp. dried root in 1 cup of water. Decoct 10–15 minutes, then steep another 30. Take ½ cup 2–3 times a day.

SYRUP: For anemia or blood deficiency, prepare a decoction of a pinch each of Yellow Dock root, Nettle, Peony root, and Red Clover with 1 tbsp. of molasses to 1 cup water. Take 1 cup 3 times a day for no more than 3 months.

TINCTURE: Take 1–2 ml. 3 times a day.

IMPORTANT: Should not be taken in combination with other diuretics, Lasix, or other drugs treating congestive heart failure or edema, as it can cause potassium depletion. Contains oxalic acid, which can interfere with calcium absorption and increase risk of kidney stones. Do not consume in large quantities or over a long period of time.

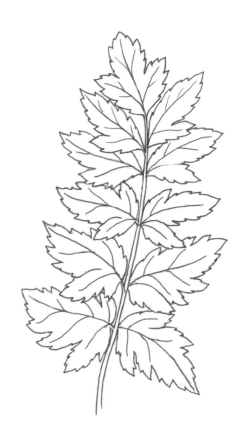

POISONOUS PLANTS

This section deals with those plants we must be extra careful to avoid, since it is very easy when wildcrafting to mistake one plant for another, and sometimes this can have dire consequences. Garden plants and poisonous plants already mentioned have not been included.

Apiaceae Family

Plants in this family are tricky to identify and include edible plants like carrot, Queen Anne's Lace, parsnip, parsley, fennel, and dill. However, there are others that can be extremely toxic and that closely resemble their edible relatives—particularly the flowers, which are usually white and in clusters arranged in umbels or umbrella-like formations. These plants contain chemicals in their sap which can cause phytophotodermatitis on the skin if touched. A good rule is: if you're not 100% sure what a plant is, leave it alone!

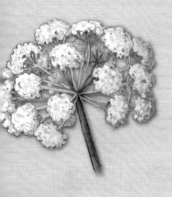

| TREATMENT |

If you accidentally touch any of these plants, immediately keep your skin away from sunlight and wash the area with cool running water. Avoid rubbing or using hot water, as this will open the pores and allow the poison to go deeper. Use a mild soap to remove any remaining residue. If there is soreness, cover the area with a cool, damp cloth. If there are open sores or blistering, apply an antibiotic cream and sterile bandage, taking care to change the bandage at least twice a day. If a large area is affected, consult your doctor.

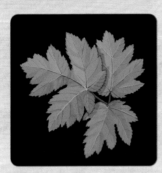

COW PARSNIP
Heracleum maximum

- Native, grows in a variety of habitats.
- Grows up to 2 metres.
- Flower umbels up to 30 cm. diameter, white.
- Leaves can be almost 60 cm. wide, hairy, and divided into 3 deeply lobed leaflets. Lobes are more rounded than those of Giant Hogweed.
- Stem does not have purple blotches like the Giant Hogweed.
- Contains furanocoumarins, which cause phytophotodermatitis, especially older plants.

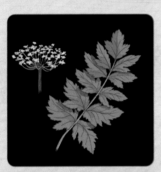

WILD PARSNIP
Pastinaca sativa

- Introduced, invasive, grows in disturbed areas, meadows.
- Grows up to 1.5 metres.
- Single green stem is smooth with few hairs and deep grooves.
- Compound leaves in pairs; sharply toothed leaflets resembling celery.
- Flowers are yellow-green and grow to 10–20 cm. across, resemble dill and fennel; single stalk with flat-topped umbel.
- Roots are edible, however great care must be taken to not touch the leaves or stalk with bare hands.

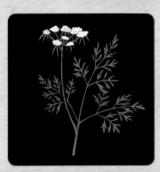

FOOL'S PARSLEY
Aethusa cynapium

- Introduced, annual or biennial.
- Hairless, smooth hollow, branched stem, up to 150 cm. in height.
- Leaves alternate, 2 or 3 times pinnate, triangular, similar to parsley but with a foul onion-like smell.
- Root shaped like a spindle, and tapered at each end.
- Flowers are white and appear in flat umbels; distinctive characteristic is 3 bracts or appendages hanging from each cluster.
- Dangerous if mistaken for parsley and ingested, for it contains poisonous alkaloids that cause burning in the digestive tract, vomiting, coldness, and even death.

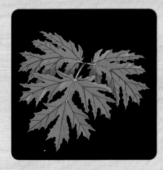

GIANT HOGWEED
Heracleum mantegazzianum

- Introduced, invasive, after 3–5 years can grow up to 5 metres high.
- Umbels are white and can be half a metre across, with over 50 rays.
- Stems thick, ridged, and hollow, with purplish blotches and stiff white bristles.
- Large lobed compound leaves with deep incisions and serrated edges.
- Causes severe phytophotodermatitis.

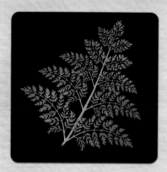

POISON HEMLOCK
Conium maculatum

- Introduced biennial, invasive, 2–3 metres tall, grows near streams and in ditches.
- Stems hairless, hollow, usually spotted with red or purple towards the base.
- Leaves are 2–4, pinnate, finely divided, triangular, and similar to a carrot's. When crushed, they emit a musty smell.
- Flowers are white and grow in loose clusters.
- All parts of this plant are poisonous; causes severe skin reactions, and when ingested can affect the nervous system, cause respiratory collapse, or even death.

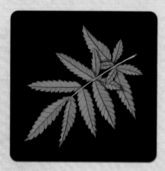

WATER HEMLOCK
Cicuta maculata

- Native perennial, .6 to 1.8 metres tall. Grows in wet areas.
- Stems are erect, mostly hollow, reddish-purple, and mostly hairless.
- Lance-shaped leaves, 2–3 times pinnate with a single leaf at the tip, coarsely toothed, with lateral veins that extend to notches between the teeth.
- Roots are fleshy, tuberous, chambered, and hollow. The yellow oily sap exuding from stem and root is foul-smelling.
- Flowers are whitish-green, with dome-shaped umbels.
- Contains cicutoxin; even small doses of the sap are lethal, causing convulsions and respiratory failure within a few hours.

Other Species to Avoid

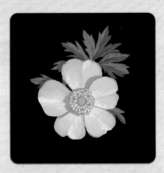

BUTTERCUP (all species)
Ranunculus
- Small perennial, about 500 species.
- Lustrous yellow flowers, cup-shaped, usually 5 petals.
- All species are poisonous if eaten fresh. The plant has an acrid taste and causes blistering in the mouth and digestive tract, bloody diarrhea or urine, and abdominal pain.
- Avoid excessive handling as it may cause contact dermatitis.
- When dried, buttercups lose their toxicity.

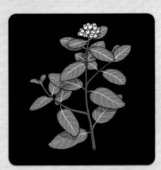

HEMP DOGBANE (INDIAN HEMP)
Apocynum cannabinum
- Native perennial resembling Milkweed. Identify Hemp Dogbane by its red stem, often branched, and smaller cluster of whitish flowers, smaller narrower leaves, and narrow seedpod.
- Grows up to 1.8 metres tall; used by Indigenous peoples to make fibre for ropes and clothing.
- Leaves are elliptical, opposite, with light-green veins.
- Flowers are small, cylindrical, and greenish-white; milky white sap in stems and leaves.
- Contains cardiac glycosides and cymarin; consumption in humans and animals may cause rapid pulse, vomiting, blue mucous membranes, weakness, convulsions.
- Treatment suggestions in animals include emetics or activated charcoal. Humans who have been poisoned should seek immediate medical help.

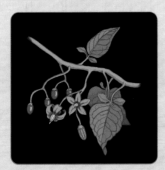

BITTERSWEET NIGHTSHADE
Solanum dulcamara
- Vine-like non-native perennial, grows up to 3 metres tall.
- Alternating heart-shaped leaves, with 2 ear-like segments at the base.
- Star-shaped purple flowers, with bright yellow stamens in the middle. Mature berries are bright red.
- Berries are toxic, and eating more than 200 is considered lethal. Particularly attractive to children as they taste a bit like tomatoes. Symptoms include diarrhea, dilated pupils, headache, vomiting, paralysis, convulsions.
- Treatment: an emetic should be administered, along with fluids.

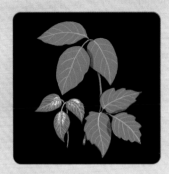

POISON IVY
Toxicodendron radicans

- Almond-shaped leaves, which are sometimes toothed, sometimes shiny, growing in groups of 3, ranging from light green to dark green, to reddish in the fall. Leaf clusters alternate on the vine, growing close to the ground or attaching to trees.
- Mainly allergenic rather than a poison, the sap contains urushiol, which causes a severe allergic reaction in most people when handled, resulting in contact dermatitis, itching, and blistering. Ingestion may cause stomach upset, but is not severe.
- Treatment: wash exposed area immediately with soap and cool water for 30 minutes; avoid spreading the oils to other parts of the body. Symptoms may be relieved by rubbing Jewelweed on the skin, applying calamine lotion, witch hazel, zinc oxide, or taking an oatmeal bath.

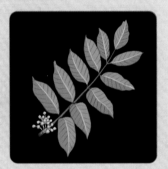

POISON SUMAC
Toxicodendron vernix

- Sparse shrub, 1.5–6 metres tall, with red stems. Thrives in wet soil, and found only in Nova Scotia and Quebec.
- Pinnate structure with 6–12 leaves growing on each side of the stem, with 1 more at the end. Each leaf is 5–10 cm. in length, almond-shaped, with wavy or smooth edges. Leaves may be orange or light green in the spring, green in summer, and red during the fall.
- Pale yellow or green flowers grow in clusters on stems separate from the leaves. These grow into green, yellow, or grey-white berries.
- Treatment is the same as for Poison Ivy.

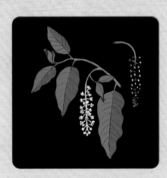

POKEWEED
Phytolacca Americana

- Native perennial, usually up to 2 metres high, and found only in New Brunswick and Quebec.
- Several stems growing out of a central taproot; stems are smooth, green to reddish, and the leaves are alternate with long petioles.
- Flowers grow in elongated racemes with bright-pink peduncles. The clusters of flowers are radially symmetric and white or greenish. Ripe berries are shiny dark purple.
- All parts are toxic to mammals, but not to birds. A violent emetic, Pokeweed causes cramps, bloody diarrhea, and/or paralysis of respiratory organs, depending on amount consumed. Plant juice may also be absorbed through the skin. If only ingested in a small amount, people or animals will recover in a day or two.

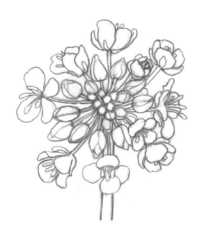

GLOSSARY

Abortifacient A substance that brings on an abortion.

Adaptogen Herbs that work on the immune and neuro-endocrine systems, increasing the body's resistance and adaptability to stress while balancing the overall physiology without being toxic, even with long-term use. Tonic, antioxidant and anti-inflammatory, not specific to any organ but helps to regulate organ and system function in general, and maintain homeostasis.

Adjuvant A substance that aids the action of a medicinal agent or medical treatment.

Alterative A medicine that favourably alters the course of an ailment and gradually restores health.

Amenorrhea Absence of menstruation, usually due to either stress, weight gain or loss, excessive exercise, cysts or tumours, hormonal imbalance, pregnancy or lactation. May be erratic, occuring for short periods of time.

Analeptic An agent that has a restorative or stimulating effect, as on the central nervous system; may act as an anticonvulsant.

Analgesic An agent that relieves pain.

Anaphrodisiac An agent that reduces one's capacity for sexual arousal.

Anodyne An agent that relieves pain or promotes comfort, usually externally.

Anthelmintic A substance that kills and expels intestinal parasitic worms.

Antibiotic An agent that inhibits the growth of or kills an organism, usually in reference to bacteria or microorganisms.

Anti-inflammatory An agent that reduces redness, heat and swelling of inflamed tissues.

Antioxidant An agent that helps protect the body from damage by free radicals, a major cause of disease and aging.

Antipyretic An agent that prevents or reduces fever.

Antilithic A substance that dissolves or reduces the size of kidney stones.

Antitussive A substance that relieves coughs.

Aperient An agent that is mildly purgative or laxative.

Astringent Remedies that cause soft tissues to pucker or draw together, usually due to the presence of tannins. They are useful for reducing irritation and inflammation and create a barrier against infection in wounds and burns. They diminish secretions, check minor bleeding, and control diarrhea. Not recommended for long-term use.

Bitters Herbs having a bitter taste which stimulate digestive juices and bile production, and subsequently increase appetite. They may also stimulate peristalsis and help repair damage in the gastrointestinal wall.

Brachycardiac An agent that makes the heart beat slower.

Carminative Soothes the gut, easing pain and causing release of stomach or intestinal gas. This action is due to the presence of volatile oils which have anti-inflammatory, antispasmodic and antimicrobial effects on the lining of the intestines.

Catarrh A condition where the mucous membranes of the nose and breathing passages are inflamed, often chronically.

Cathartic A purgative or laxative causing evacuation of the bowels.

Cholagogue An agent that increases the flow of bile from the gallbladder, which in turn facilitates fat digestion and works as a natural laxative. Should not be used with toxic liver disorders, acute viral hepatitis, painful gallstones or other acute liver problems.

Decoction A herbal preparation of roots or woody plant material boiled in water.

Demulcent Herbs which tend to become slimy in water and work to form a barrier on irritated tissues, soothing inflammation of the mucous membranes. They reduce irritation all through the digestive tract, easing muscle spasms and sensitivity to gastric acids, as well as easing coughs, sore throat, and pain in the bladder and urinary systems.

Depurative An agent that has a purifying effect.

Diaphoretic An agent that usually works by relaxing the sweat glands and inducing a greater outward flow of blood, thereby increasing the amount of perspiration. This rids the body of offensive materials and aids the immune and endocrine systems.

Diuretic An agent that helps the body get rid of excess fluids by increasing urine flow, helping with a wide range of disorders where too much fluid accumulates in the tissues (edema).

Dropsy An old-fashioned term for edema or lymph congestion.

Dysmenorrhea Painful menstruation with cramping, due to a variety of underlying causes.

Edema A build-up of fluids in the tissues causing swelling.

Emetic An agent that induces vomiting.

Emmenagogue An agent that regulates and stimulates normal menstruation, as well as having a toning effect on the female reproductive system.

Expectorant An agent that facilitates the expulsion of phlegm from the respiratory tract by irritating and stimulating the bronchioles to liquefy and move thick sputum upwards so it can be cleared more easily by coughing, or by relaxing and loosening thinner mucous as in a dry cough.

Febrifuge An agent that relieves fever.

Galactagogue An agent that promotes the flow of milk.

Hemagogue An agent that promotes the flow of blood.

Hemostatic An agent that controls or stops bleeding.

Hepatic A herbal remedy that supports the liver by toning, strengthening, and in some cases detoxifying and increasing the flow of bile, which in turn affects the entire digestive system.

Hypnotic A herb that promotes sleep and has a relaxing effect on the nervous system.

Hypertensive An agent that causes a rise in blood pressure.

Hypotensive An agent that reduces elevated blood pressure.

Infusion A herbal preparation made by soaking it in hot or cold water to be drunk as a tea.

Lactifuge An agent that increases the flow of milk in lactating women.

Leukorrhea Thick, white vaginal discharge.

Menorrhagia Excessive menstrual bleeding; in younger women usually as a result of fibroids, tumours, polyps, endometriosis, or blood-clotting problems; in older women typically caused by erratic hormones due to premenopause.

Mucilaginous Containing a gel-like, slimy substance called mucilage which can be helpful in soothing inflammation.

Nervine An agent that has a beneficial effect on the nervous system. Depending on the plant, this can work as a tonic, which repairs damage to the nervous system in cases of trauma or stress; as a relaxant, which eases anxiety and relaxes the peripheral nerves, muscles and organs of the body; or as a stimulant, which helps enhance vitality where the body is sluggish.

Parturient A substance which aids in the birthing process.

Poultice A warm mass of plant material, or a cloth wrapped in plant material, which is applied to the skin to cause a medicinal action.

Purgative An agent that acts as a strong laxative, cleansing the bowel, often with cramping and pain.

Rubefacient Causing localized reddening of the skin.

Saponin A compound in some plants that has a foaming or soapy action when shaken with water.

Scrofula Swellings of the lymph glands in the neck, caused by tuberculosis.

Styptic A substance that slows or stops bleeding by contracting the blood vessels; astringent.

Stomachic An agent that aids the stomach and digestion.

Tincture A herbal medicine prepared by soaking plant material in alcohol, cider vinegar, or glycerine over a period of time and then straining, in order to extract the medicinal compounds.

Vermifuge An agent that rids the body of worms (anthelmintic).

Vulnerary A remedy that promotes healing of wounds.

BIBLIOGRAPHY

Boxer, Arabella and Philippa Back. *The Herb Book*. London: Octopus Books Limited, 1981.

Buhner, Stephen Harrod. *Sacred Plant Medicine: The Wisdom in Native American Herbalism*. Rochester, VT: Bear & Company, 2006.

Bunney, Sarah. *The Illustrated Encyclopedia of Herbs, Their Medicinal and Culinary Uses*. London: Chancellor Press, 1992.

Burke, Nancy. *The Modern Herbal Primer, A Simple Guide to the Magic and Medicine of 100 Healing Herbs*. Alexandria, Virginia: Time-Life Books (Old Farmer's Almanac Home Library), 2000.

Castleman, Michael. *The Healing Herbs, The Ultimate Guide to the Curative Power of Nature's Medicines*. Emmaus, Pennsylvania: Rodale Press, 1991.

Clough, Katherine. *Wildflowers of Prince Edward Island*. Charlottetown, PEI: Ragweed Press, 1995.

Duke, James A. *The Green Pharmacy*. Emmaus, Pennsylvania: Rodale Press, 1997.

Foster, Steven and Rebecca L. Johnson. *Desk Reference to Nature's Medicine*. Washington, DC: National Geographic Society, 2006.

Foster, Steven and James A. Duke. *Eastern/Central Medicinal Plants and Herbs of Eastern and Central North America*. New York: Houghton Mifflin Company (Peterson Field Guide Series), 2000.

Grieve, Maud. *A Modern Herbal*. London: Tiger Books International, 1973 (Originally published in 1931).

Hoffmann, David. *The Complete Illustrated Holistic Herbal*. London: Element (An Imprint of Harper Collins), 2002.

Lacey, Laurie. *Mi'kmaq Medicines, Remedies and Recollections*. Halifax, NS: Nimbus Publishing, 2012.

MacKinnon, Andrew. *Edible & Medicinal Plants of Canada*. Edmonton, Alberta: Lone Pine Publishing, Co-published by Lone Pine Media Productions (BC), 2009.

Pahlow, Mannfried. *Healing Plants*. Hauppauge, NY: Barron's Educational Series, Inc., 1993.

Redfield, Edmund. *Wildflowers of the Maritimes: A Guide to Identifying 150 of the Region's Wild Plants*. Halifax, NS: Nimbus Publishing, 2016.

Reader's Digest. *Magic and Medicine of Plants*. Pleasantville, New York: Reader's Digest Association, Inc., 1989.

Scott, Peter J. *Edible Plants of Atlantic Canada*. Portugal Cove-St. Philip's, Newfoundland and Labrador: Boulder Publications, 2010.

Tierra, Michael. *The Way of Herbs*. New York: Pocket Books (Simon and Shuster), 1998.

Vermeulen, Nico. *The Complete Encyclopedia of Herbs*. Lisse, The Netherlands: Rebo Publishers, 1998.

Walker, Marilyn. *Wild Plants of Eastern Canada*. Halifax, NS: Nimbus Publishing, 2008.

Wood, Matthew. *The Earthwise Herbal Repertory*. Berkeley, California: North Atlantic Books, 2016.

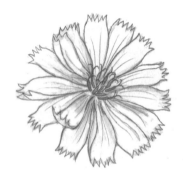